HOMEOPATHY

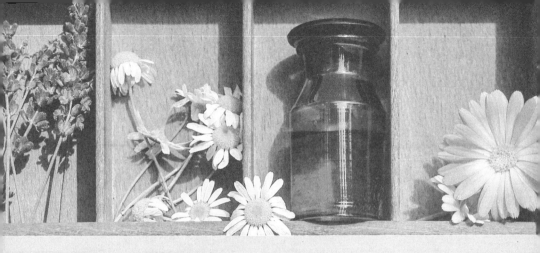

HOMEOPATHY

THE COMPLETE GUIDE TO
NATURAL
REMEDIES

ALBERT-CLAUDE QUEMOUN, PhD
with SOPHIE PENSA

STERLING ETHOS
New York

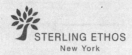

STERLING ETHOS
New York

An Imprint of Sterling Publishing Co., Inc.
1166 Avenue of the Americas
New York, NY 10036

ISBN 978-1-4549-2637-5

Library of Congress Cataloging-in-Publication Data
Names: Quemoun, Albert-Claude, author. | Pensa, Sophie, author.
Title: Homeopathy : the complete guide to natural remedies / by Albert-Claude
    Quemoun, with Sophie Pensa.
Other titles: Homéopathie. English
Description: New York : Sterling Ethos, 2019.
Identifiers: LCCN 2019004413 | ISBN 9781454926375 (paperback)
Subjects: LCSH: Homeopathy. | Herbs--Therapeutic use. | BISAC: HEALTH &
    FITNESS / Homeopathy. | HEALTH & FITNESS / Herbal Medications. | HEALTH &
    FITNESS / Alternative Therapies.
Classification: LCC RX71 .Q8413 2019 | DDC 615.5/32--dc23
LC record available at https://lccn.loc.gov/2019004413

Distributed in Canada by Sterling Publishing Co., Inc.
c/o Canadian Manda Group, 664 Annette Street
Toronto, Ontario M6S 2C8, Canada
Distributed in the United Kingdom by GMC Distribution Services
Castle Place, 166 High Street, Lewes, East Sussex BN7 1XU, England
Distributed in Australia by NewSouth Books
University of New South Wales, Sydney, NSW 2052, Australia

For information about custom editions, special sales, and premium and corporate purchases,
please contact Sterling Special Sales at 800-805-5489 or specialsales@sterlingpublishing.com.

Interior design by Sharon Jacobs and Nancy Singer
Cover design by David Ter-Avanesyan
Cover photograph by Marina Lohrbach/Getty Images

Manufactured in Canada

2 4 6 8 10 9 7 5 3 1

sterlingpublishing.com

To the memory of my father, and to my mother,
who showed me a great deal of affection.

To my teachers, who knew how to inspire in me their passion
for a form of treatment that was so effective and nontoxic.

To my colleagues and friends who were doctors, pharmacists,
veterinarians, and dentists and who encouraged me.

To the universities.

To the lecturers at Institut Homéopathique Scientifique
(Homeopathic Scientific Institute). Centre Homéopathique
de France (French Center for Homeopathy), Institut National
Homéopathique Français (French National Homeopathic Institute).
Société Française d'Homéopathie (French Homeopathic Society),
and Société Médicale de Biothérapie (Medical Society of Biotherapy).

To the researchers at Institut National de la Santé et de Recherche
Médicale (French National Institute of Health and Medical Research;
INSERM) who validated my ideas.

To my family and friends.

To my collaborators.

To the editor and editorial team, who have a lot of patience and have
supported me in expressing my views.

To Dr. Olivier Rabanes, who reviewed and corrected the historical details.

To Dr. Florine Boukhobza, who proofread what I wrote.

CONTENTS

PREFACE

HOMEOPATHY IS AN EFFECTIVE FORM OF MEDICINE. ITS greatest advantage is that it is nontoxic and does not cause side effects. But for a beginner, it can sometimes be complicated to use.

This book is a practical guide intended for:

- Professionals starting in practice

- Families who need practical advice while waiting for the doctor

- All those who wish to understand the rudiments of homeopathy

You will find a wealth of information suited to your needs throughout this book and advice that is very easy to put into practice, with detailed indexes to enable you to find the information you are looking for as quickly as possible. This book is also a reference manual that will help you discover the subtleties of homeopathy and its incomparable advantages, but also its difficulties and occasional pitfalls.

Knowledge of homeopathy will enable you to use the remedies that fit your ailments, your personality, and your reactions, whether physical, mental, or emotional. You will discover a type of medicine in which each person who is ill is treated as unique and is questioned and treated with care and attention. Homeopathy treats each person in a specific and special way with the remedy that suits them at every moment of their life. It can even make the task easier with complex remedies prepared specifically for the patient or already available on the market.

It is often necessary to consult a doctor for a detailed diagnosis as well as for such things as lab tests, X-rays, MRIs, or other scans. Using conventional medicines is sometimes necessary, even after taking into account their often toxic effects. Most often, homeopathic techniques are complementary; when homeopathy is not enough to cure a problem, it can help to support standard allopathic treatment.

I have devoted my life to homeopathy and would like to share my knowledge and experience with you. I want this book to be your guide and be useful to you.

—ALBERT-CLAUDE QUEMOUN

CHAPTER 1

INTRODUCTION TO HOMEOPATHY

Homeopathy:
from the Greek *hómoios* (similar) and *páthos* (suffering).

CHRISTIAN FRIEDRICH SAMUEL HAHNEMANN, THE FOUNDING FATHER OF HOMEOPATHY

S AMUEL HAHNEMANN WAS A GERMAN DOCTOR FROM Saxony, where he set up in practice in 1779 at the age of twenty-four. He was brilliant and independent and was soon disappointed with the medical practice of his time, which he judged to be ineffective. In 1790, he decided to devote his time to research based on experimentation, which was a completely revolutionary method at that time.

Hahnemann wanted to test medicines and substances on individuals who were in good health to assess their effects.

First, he experimented on himself, taking *Cinchona* bark to assess its impact. This was a medicine recently brought back from South America and used to treat fevers, but *Cinchona* was still not well understood, and its side effects had been poorly assessed.

THE REDISCOVERY OF SIMILITUDE

It was in translating *Materia Medica* by William Cullen that Hahnemann realized that *Cinchona*, which was then used to treat fever, could cause a fever to develop, similar to the one it had treated, if it was administered for too long. Hahnemann took *Cinchona* when he was in good health and was surprised to find that he started to suffer from fevers, palpitations, and fatigue. He observed that he was producing the symptoms that this medicine was supposed to cure. He had just rediscovered the principle of similitude, already described by Hippocrates: "By similar things a disease is produced and through the application of the like is cured."

After repeating the same experiment on some friends, he deduced from it the law upon which homeopathy was founded: to cure an illness, it is necessary to administer a remedy that would cause similar symptoms in a healthy person to those of the illness that the sick person is suffering from.

THE INNOVATION OF THE INFINITESIMAL

Hahnemann continued his research, convinced that the results he had observed with *Cinchona* were transferable to other products. He experimented in this way on healthy individuals to find the effects of many other substances and discover their curative properties.

He also researched ways of limiting the side effects of these substances and perfected a completely original method of production: the infinitesimal, a method that consisted of extracting the active principles of a substance and greatly diluting them, so that the patient ingested only minute doses.

THE BIRTH OF HOMEOPATHY

In 1796, after six years of research and experimentation, he published his conclusions in Christoph Hufeland's *Journal de médecine pratique (Journal of Practical Medicine)*, the most important medical journal at the time, with the heading: "Treatise on a new principle for revealing the curative properties of medicinal substances, followed by some observations on the principles accepted up until the present time."

This is the official birth of homeopathy, and it was also the beginning of the calvary of Samuel Hahnemann. Envied, contested, criticized, and detested by his colleagues and the Académie de Médecine (Academy of Medicine), he went through many court cases and humiliations—and a number of successes and cures.

HAHNEMANN'S HERITAGE

He never ceased, however, to refine his discoveries and, in 1810, he published the first edition of his *Organon of the Rational Art of Healing*. There would be five more of these, the last being posthumous.

Before his death in 1843 in Paris, with his second wife at his side (a French woman, Mélanie d'Hervilly), he wrote *Materia Medica Pura* and *The Chronic Diseases*. While he had obtained brilliant results with acute conditions, chronic diseases presented an obstacle, and he realized that the patient should be treated differently in these two situations. This is one issue I shall address in more depth in this book, expanding on deep-acting treatments, diatheses, and constitutions.

THE FUTURE OF HOMEOPATHY

Hahnemann thus provided a solid base, which even today is being perfected and improved, for hundreds of thousands of doctors who practice homeopathy throughout the world. In fact, it is up to the homeopaths of today to unite to continue the scientific work of Hahnemann and definitively aim to develop a modern type of medicine for the future.

THE MAIN PRINCIPLES OF HOMEOPATHY

The law of similars

This is the basic rule of homeopathy, spelled out by Hippocrates and experienced by Hahnemann: like cures like. The symptoms of an illness can be cured by a substance that causes the same symptoms in a healthy person. For example, when a bee stings you, initially you feel pain, followed by edema and a burning sensation, which can be soothed by applying cold compresses. By analogy, if you have a burning pain in a joint, with edema, which feels better with cold compresses, you could think of using Apis mellifica (a medicine made from bees) to treat it.

The law of the infinitesimal dose

Even in small doses, active substances can produce unpleasant side effects in the patient or be too toxic to be ingested without danger. Successive dilution of the products, to the point of obtaining infinitesimal doses, can avoid this problem. Many different methods of preparation make it possible, ultimately, to produce infinitesimal doses in various ways.

Totality of symptoms

Within the context of an illness, the homeopathic doctor does not take into account only one single symptom, but many. A simple attack of nausea does not sum up a pathology.

The practitioner also takes into account the person's behavior and psychological symptoms. In homeopathy, you would not prescribe a remedy for pain, but for a person who is suffering, depending on the way the person suffers. Each of us can react differently to the same symptom.

Let us take the case of pain due to muscle trauma or muscle contraction.

- If the pain is due to the flu or a sports injury, and if the patient suffers from the slightest movement and even their bed feels too hard, you would prescribe Arnica montana.

- If the pain improves with rest or when you press the muscle, or if the patient spontaneously lies on the painful side, you would choose Bryonia alba.

- If, on the contrary, movement helps the patient, you would choose Rhus toxicodendron.

- If the patient suffers in silence, shuts themselves in their room, and seems stoic, as if they were oblivious to the pain, you would advise Sepia.

- If, on the contrary, the suffering causes tears and the person seeks consolation, feels better in the fresh air, and is timid, you will give Pulsatilla.

To sum up, you do not treat an isolated symptom, but a number of symptoms in a person whose behavior you perceive as a totality, while in conventional medicine (allopathy) you would be content to prescribe a painkiller.

Concepts of terrain, profile, and behavior

Faced with the same pathology, people who are sick behave differently, and you can imagine their reactions by observing them in their everyday life when they are healthy and feel well. This attitude is a valuable indication of their reaction when they are ill.

To be able to assess this behavior better, you have to understand the individual as a whole. This includes their physical aspect (their constitution) as well as their organic way of reacting to the illness (their diathesis). These two aspects constitute what is referred to as the terrain of the person. The person's approach to everyday life is also taken into account. All this information makes it possible to define the patient profile.

constitution + diathesis (reaction to the illness) = terrain

terrain + behavior = profile

THE CONSTITUTIONS

Are you square, round, slim, asymmetric, fat, or tall? Whatever the case, your constitution can make it possible to anticipate specific pathology or particular forms of pathology adopted by the same illness, which you can also predict and preempt.

Carbonic constitution

Their physique: They are brachymorphic (short and broad); they have short fingers, toes, and limbs; wide palms; and the powerful physique of a strong worker. If you caricatured them, you would think of sumo wrestlers or bulldogs. These people do not do things very fast, but they finish everything that they have begun. They start slowly but finish brilliantly, like the tortoise in the fable. They very much like to eat and sometimes eat everything.

Their pathologies: They tend to be retentive and not eliminate well, particularly if they do not exercise or if they are sedentary. They are subject to weight gain, excess uric acid, hypertension, physical or general slowing down, rheumatism aggravated by excess weight, and so on.

Fluoric constitution

Their physique: They are asymmetric, their spine is not completely straight, they are hypermobile, their arms have a tendency to go backward, their fingers tend to be perpendicular to the palm of the hand, and their skeleton may be deformed. If you caricatured them, you would think of Quasimodo or a dachshund. Their tissues are fragile.

Their pathologies: Their skeletal asymmetry makes them subject to sciatica, dorsal and lumbar back pain, asymmetry in teeth (which causes cavities), weakness and prolapse of organs in women due to their hyperlax ligaments, and dilation of their veins, causing poor circulation and varicose ulcers.

Phosphoric constitution

Their physique: They are willowy—they grow up too fast and are rather thin. If you caricatured them, you would think of Don Quixote or a greyhound. They get off to a flying start, like the hare in the fable, but although they are quick to ignite, they are exhausted equally quickly and have difficulty in finishing what they have started. At school, phosphoric children achieve excellent results in the first term but run out of steam over the course of the year. They are passionate and have a lot of ideas, all of which they want to implement.

Their pathologies: Being so tall means that they suffer from tension in the dorsal vertebrae and, as they have a tendency to stoop, this only exacerbates this problem. They should avoid professions in which it is necessary to be in a stooping position the entire day, such as dentistry. They are subject to respiratory problems, suffer from poor digestion, physical deterioration, and demineralization.

Sulfuric constitution

Their physique: They are of average build. They like to live well, often sweat, and have a ruddy complexion and clammy hands.

Their pathologies: As a rule, they don't get ill, but as time goes on, they have more problems with elimination and may develop illnesses associated with retention. Skin conditions may alter-nate with internal problems.

Combinations (composite constitution)

An individual can present characteristics of several constitutions: one may find carbo-fluorics (stocky with an asymmetry of the skeleton), phospho-fluorics (tall and asymmetric), and so on.

THE DIATHESES

While the constitution doesn't change and is inherent to each individual, the diatheses (reactions to the illness) develop in time and space. There are four main diatheses, defined by the behavior of the person when confronted with their ailments.

Psoric diathesis

Behavior: Psoric people eliminate profusely in a centrifugal manner, from the interior to the exterior. Their skin is not always clear because, as a result of eliminating to the exterior, there can be small spots, acne, boils, or eczema. Psoric people often suffer from itching, aggravated by contact with water and the heat of the bed. Thermoregulation is difficult (either they are too hot, as with the Sulfur picture, or too cold, like the profile for Arsenicum album). They have a tendency toward parasitic conditions, and they are often the people who attract mosquitoes. They have alternating skin and internal symptoms. These people are mostly optimistic and extroverted.

Their pathologies are aggravated when elimination stops. It is particularly important not to block it. You should avoid, for example, stopping a nosebleed in a psoric person with hypertension, because that may be serving as a safety valve. It is better to have a simple hemorrhage from the nose than a brain hemorrhage or a stroke.

But you may also observe alternation over time. A person may suffer from asthma attacks at night and feel fine when they wake up. This patient fights their illness themselves and regulates their pathology according to time of day, the moment, and by producing successive symptoms. This is how nutritional intoxication resolves itself in a psoric person: by a case of diarrhea or vomiting or a skin eruption, and all is forgotten. This is completely the opposite of a sycotic person, who will not be able to eliminate and whose state of health will be aggravated by this situation of intoxication.

The remedies: Many remedies are suitable for a psoric constitution, including Sulfur, Arsenicum album, Nux vomica, or Psorinum.

Sycotic diathesis

Behavior: Instead of elimination to the exterior like psorics, sycotics have a tendency toward concentration and centripetal elimination toward the interior. Consequently, they are subject to water retention, warts, condylomata, and fibroids in women.

This could be the case with a psoric person who has difficulty eliminating following a vaccination, for example, or a person on cortisone, who then becomes a victim of water retention and weight gain.

The health of a sycotic person is usually aggravated by humidity but improved with slow movement. They often suffer from ear, nose, and throat conditions or urogenital problems after vaccination or a sexually transmitted disease. They can have joint problems.

Generally speaking, sycotic people are introverts. Sometimes characterized by obsessions, they can have a tendency toward depression.

The remedies: Many remedies are suitable for a sycotic reaction: Thuja occidentalis, Natrum sulphuricum, Dulcamara, Rhus toxicodendron.

As they age, some sycotic people are exposed to dehydration and so to withering of the skin: these are dry sycotics. Their joints and limbs could retract. Their state improves on contact with humidity. The remedy for them is Causticum.

Tubercular diathesis

Behavior: Tubercular people tend to lose weight even if they eat normally. They are frequently subject to pulmonary or respiratory problems. They can suffer from venous stasis and demineralization. They are often cold, except when they have hyperthyroid problems (in this case, they are always hot).

Where elimination is concerned, tubercular people are between psoric and sycotic: neither expulsion to the exterior nor retention, but a mucus discharge (urogenital, vaginal, respiratory). Elimination is slow. Tubercular people are subject to repeated colds and strep throat. With time, their resistance to disease diminishes.

Their state improves with slow movement, such as walking.

The remedies: Several remedies are suitable for a tubercular reaction: Phosphorus, Pulsatilla, Natrum muriaticum, Iodum, Arsenicum iodatum.

Syphilitic Diathesis

Behavior: Syphilitics have a fragile appearance. They are often agitated and may suffer from cirrhosis, conditions due to the destruction of cells or tissues, ulceration, chancres, and bone problems. Their state improves in the mountains and is aggravated by the sea and during the night. They can be plagued by irrational fear of germs and wash their hands continually, meticulously disinfecting the smallest sores.

The remedies: Several remedies are suitable for a syphilitic constitution: Syphilinum, Mercurius solubilis, Argentum nitricum, Aurum metallicum, Lachesis, Sulphuricum acidum, Fluoricum acidum.

Progression from one diathesis to another

A psoric person may become sycotic, especially if you block their eliminations. A sycotic can become syphilitic if they begin to have ulcerations or lose weight.

ONE DIATHESIS, ONE TREATMENT

Let us take the case of a venous pathology. The psoric presents with varicose eczema, the sycotic has retention in the legs (theirs are "like fence posts"), the tubercular person suffers from small varicosities, and the syphilitic from varicose ulcers.

You, therefore, do not treat these people in the same way, in spite of the original problem being identical. Even if all of them took the same venous tonic, you would give each the deep remedy based on their constitution.

PROFILES

To understand the person's profile, you have to observe them as a whole. The profile takes into account constitution and diathesis, but also everyday behavior: are they agitated, slow, sleepy, intelligent? Are they better lying in bed or when physically active? Are they extroverted or closed? Are they better with movement or rest, aggravated or not by being consoled, and so on?

As opposed to constitutions or diatheses, which form groups with general characteristics, the profile determines the unique remedy for that person. With homeopathy, you find a treatment that is not only therapeutic but can be used prophylactically.

On page 233 you will find a detailed definition of a great many profiles and their indications.

What is a homeopathic remedy made of?

Homeopathic remedies are made of active substances from three great kingdoms: vegetable, mineral, and animal.

THE VEGETABLE KINGDOM

The vegetable kingdom provides 60 percent of the sources for homeopathic remedies. You can use the whole plant (*Arnica* from the mountains for Arnica montana or the fungus puffball for Bovista) or only one part (the tobacco leaf for Tabacum, the bark of red *Cinchona* for China rubra, the *Thuja* branch for Thuja occidentalis).

THE MINERAL KINGDOM

These can be used in the form of simple elements (gold for Aurum metallicum, silver for Argentum metallicum), salts (silver nitrate for Argentum nitricum) or natural complex salts (sea salt for Natrum muriaticum), or products defined by the method of production (Mercurius solubilis).

THE ANIMAL KINGDOM (LIVING THINGS)

Organic substances are derived mainly from pigs, ducks, or rabbits. They are subjected to strict viral security controls, which have been even stricter since the mad cow disease crisis. Certain species, like cows, sheep, and goats, are no longer used out of concern for transmission of viruses.

They may originate in an organ (kidney for Renin, liver for Hepatin, brain for Cerebellum), from the whole animal (the bee for Apis mellifica, the red ant for Formica rufa), from a secretion of the animal (the dried ink for Sepia, snake venom for Lachesis, viper venom for Vipera redi), from a bacterial substance or toxins (culture of inactivated staphylococcus for Staphylococcinum), serums, or vaccines (the flu vaccine for Influenzinum).

They can also be of human origin. Five of them have renewed authorization for the market since 1999, in sterilized form (syphilis chancre for Syphilinum, measles secretion for Morbillinum, mange lesion for Psorinum, sample taken from the throat of a person with whooping cough for Pertussinum, urethral discharge from a subject with gonorrhea (blennorrhagia) who has not had antibiotic treatment for Medorrhinum).

How is a homeopathic remedy made?

THE HAHNEMANNIAN METHOD

Samuel Hahnemann was the first to define the production process for homeopathic remedies.

Production of mother tincture

If they can be macerated in a mixture of alcohol and water, the primary materials of the remedy (whether these are vegetal, chemical, or organic) are first crushed or reduced to powder. They are then immersed in a mixture of alcohol and distilled water, in proportions of a tenth part of the active substance to nine-tenths of solvent.

After maceration for a minimum of two weeks, the liquid is pressed and filtered in order to obtain a mother tincture. The latter is very active, even toxic. This is the case for Aconite, Belladonna, and Hemlock. To avoid side effects, it is necessary to dilute the mother tincture.

The necessity of dilution

The mother tincture is diluted many times in the solvent. The process of dilution does not make the diluted substance less effective. The more the mother tincture is diluted, the weaker the doses and the less toxic the substance. Consequently, it does not have side effects, but it remains equally effective. It just acts over a longer time period or on more general symptoms.

DH and CH

Hahnemann defined two methods of dilution: the centesimal (1 drop of mother tincture to 99 drops of solvent—which is known as CH, Hahnemannian centesimal), and the decimal (1 drop of mother tincture to 9 drops of solvent—which is known as DH, Hahnemannian decimal).

Successive dilutions

As a general rule, you use successive dilutions.

Shake at least 100 times on each transfer.

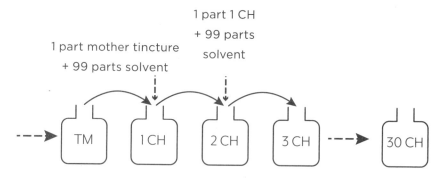

1 part 1 CH
+ 99 parts
solvent

1 part mother tincture
+ 99 parts solvent

TM   1 CH   2 CH   3 CH   30 CH

After diluting the mother tincture in 99 drops of solvent, you take 1 drop from this preparation to redilute it in another bottle with the same quantity of solvent, and repeat as often as necessary. Between each dilution, the preparation is potentized, or succussed vigorously (shaken, with at least 100 agitations at each stage), which activates the strength of the remedy.

POTENTIZATION

Potentization is shaking the preparation hard to activate the strength of the remedy. This process, now carried out mechanically in a laboratory, modifies the physical structure of the solution, which explains its efficacy, according to the latest research.

The number and the method of dilution are systematically recorded on the remedy labels. In this way, if you have a tube of Arnica montana 7 CH, you know that your remedy was manufactured from mountain arnica, macerated and then diluted seven times, successively, on a scale of 1 to 100 (or a concentration of 10^{-14}, according to the Hahnemannian technique).

MATHEMATICS LESSON

Knowing that $1/10 = 10^{-1}$, that $1/100 = 10^{-2}$, and that $1/1,000 = 10^{-3}$, a concentration of 10^{-14} is equivalent to 1/100,000,000,000,000, or a dilution of the active substance by one per one hundred thousand billion.

Trituration

As far as insoluble substances are concerned, the trituration technique is used instead of dilution. This entails mixing and kneading the active substance with lactose for about an hour. One gram of the active substance to 9 grams of lactose makes it possible to obtain a first DH. With 1 gram of the active substance to 99 grams of lactose, it is possible to obtain a first CH.

THE KORSAKOVIAN METHOD

The Russian count Simon Nicolaievitch von Korsakoff, a contemporary of Hahnemann's, then perfected a second technique of dilution, called Korsakovian, or "single bottle preparation," represented by a K. The emphasis is more on potentization than dilution, contrary to the Hahnemannian method.

In fact, after the first dilution, the solution is potentized and then completely discarded. The same bottle is then refilled with solvent, the traces of the preceding dilution on the sides of the bottle being sufficient to ensure the continuity of the process. The measure of efficacy of the remedy is in the number of potentizations undergone by the solution. An Arnica montana 10,000 K is, therefore, a remedy that has been successively potentized 1,000,000 times, in 10,000 repeated operations.

HAHNEMANN'S 50 MILLESIMAL METHOD

The third method, symbolized by LM, is especially for people who are too sensitive to any dilution or to a considerable number of succussions or potentizations.

It is enough to take a pillule of a classic dose, dissolve it in a drop of water, and add this to 100 drops of water and alcohol mixture.

One drop of this solution is then enough to potentize 500 microgranules. You thus obtain a dilution to 50 thousandths (from one dilution to the hundredth for 500 microglobules).

In the remedy name, the number of successive cycles is indicated before the LM (3 LM, 4 LM, and so on).

COMPARISON OF THE DIFFERENT DILUTIONS		
Hahnemannian decimal scale	Hahnemannian centesimal scale	Korsakovian scale
1 DH		
2 DH	1 CH	
3 DH		
4 DH	2 CH	
6 DH	3 CH	
10 DH	5 CH	30 K
14 DH	7 CH	200 K
18 DH	9 CH	5,000 K
24 DH	12 CH	
30 DH	15 CH	
48 DH	24 CH	
60 DH	30 CH	

Note that the equivalents are only exact in theory, but according to the dilution techniques, these are no longer the same products, in particular because of their degree of potentization. In fact, a 7 CH, for example, has been succussed 7 × 100 times, while a 200 K has been succussed 200 × 100 times, or 20,000 times.

How does the homeopathic remedy work?

The way that homeopathic remedies work is not yet completely understood. The very high dilution of the products does not suggest a classic chemical action.

TRANSMISSION OF INFORMATION

The importance of potentization in the manufacturing process of the remedy makes one think that the base substance must be able to transmit information, the nature of which is not precisely known, to the solvent. Is it physical, energetic, electromagnetic? Does it relate to the corporeal memory? Or is it something completely different? There are a great many hypotheses, but none has yet been proved. You can be sure that the information travels, that it has the characteristics of the base substance, and that it makes it possible to initiate the healing process. Medical practice demonstrates it every day; it remains up to researchers to explain it.

TEACHING EXPERIMENTATION

During the work I have been able to carry out with INSERM at the Saint-Antoine Hospital, in collaboration with William Rostène and his assistant Marie-Noëlle Montagne, it has been demonstrated that a homeopathic dilution can act on a receptor and displace certain neurotransmitters.

Imagine a brain receptor blocked by a product, like the lock of a car door obstructed by chewing gum. We have marked this product (the chewing gum) using a radioactive substance whose path in the human body can be easily followed. Then imagine that in allopathic medicine one molecule is sufficient to combat the product (like a good chewing gum solvent). We have been able to prove that the administration of a homeopathic remedy made from this molecule gets rid of the product, as the solvent gets rid of the chewing gum. And because the product is radioactively marked, we can follow its path, thanks to a technique called autoradiography.

THE WAVELENGTH OF THE PRODUCT

The homeopathic remedy, which is very diluted, no longer contains any active molecule of the original substance. But it works. It could be that the wavelength of the homeopathic product is the active principle. Even though we find ourselves again in an area that is hypothetical, most researchers who work on infinitesimal (very diluted) doses see their results converge toward the same hypothesis: the transmission of information from the molecule coming from a transmitter, and the receiving of this information by a receptor. That is Jacques Benveniste's theory.

The right transmitter and the right receiver must still be found, without being disrupted by other concurrent or interfering transmissions. And it is still a wide-open field of research.

The state of homeopathy in France

Homeopathic remedies were initially made by the homeopaths themselves. Then, as practitioners observed the efficacy of homeopathy, they argued for standards and legislation for specific and rigorous methods of manufacture.

THE FIRST PHARMACOPEIAS

After years of effort, started at the time of Hahnemann himself, manufacturing was delegated to pharmacists, leading to the first pharmacopeias. These works specify the precise methods of production for the remedies, as stipulated by doctors and homeopathic practitioners: Hahnemann, Jenichen, and Korsakov from 1834; Jahr in 1841 and then reedited in collaboration with Catellan in 1853; Weber in 1854; Écalle, Delpech, and Peuvrier in 1898.

COMPETITION BETWEEN LABORATORIES

With the development of standards for selection and quality control of the primary materials, the pharmacopeia developed: in the 1980s, thirteen laboratories in France specialized in the production of homeopathic remedies. There are only five today, and it is becoming more and more difficult for them to survive. One can imagine that industrial competition will lead, in the end, to a merging or outright elimination of certain laboratories.

HOMEOPATHY IN EUROPE

Today, the European pharmacopeia has opened its doors to homeopathy, and Europe is legislating in this field, which does not by itself remove all the obstacles to a clear definition of homeopathic remedies.

While manufacturing seems to have been perfected where the Hahnemannian dilutions are concerned, the production of mother tinctures still does not seem precisely defined. As an example of this, the concentration that is called mother tincture in France is different from that in Germany, the French equivalent to the first dilution in Germany (1 DH or 1 X), which throws off all the equivalents for the weak dilutions of remedies between the German and the French ones.

LEGAL DEFINITION

At the moment, European legislation defines homeopathic remedies as having to comply with a number of conditions (L 311/77, article 14, Official Journal of the European Community [Journal Officiel des Communautés Européennes], of 11/28/2001):

- Oral or external route of administration.

- An absence of particular therapeutic indication on the label or in any other information relating to the remedy.

- A degree of dilution guaranteeing the harmlessness of the remedy; in particular, a remedy may not contain either more than 1 part per 10,000 of mother tincture, or more than 1/100th of the smallest dose of an active substance that in an allopathic medicine would require a prescription.

HOMEOPATHY IN FRANCE

It was not until 1965 that homeopathic remedies were legally manufactured in France, using the Hahnemannian technique.

Single mother tinctures and single or complex remedies in Hahnemannian dilution were, from that year, reimbursed at 65 percent by French social security. Now, they are only reimbursed at 35 percent, although they represent only 1 percent of spending on medicines in France.

Furthermore, many isotherapies can no longer be used, such as those made from the secretions of the person who is ill to cure their illness, as with all the remedies sourced from substances of human origin. This is a great pity because these remedies were remarkably effective. Urinary isotherapy, for example, had excellent results for cystitis.

Saliva isotherapy is also not allowed, in the name of therapeutic safety. But how can anyone imagine that you could toxify yourself with your own saliva, especially in infinitesimal dilution? Does anyone forbid us from swallowing our own saliva when we are ill?

In this way the number of remedies authorized in France is being progressively reduced, the development of laboratories is being curtailed, and the rate of reimbursement is being cut back. It affects the very credibility of homeopathy. Today, the practice of this medicine has been damaged by incompetent people who know nothing about homeopathy and abolish remarkable remedies, and also by homeopaths who do not know how to defend their specialty.

RESEARCH

At the same time, the laboratories continue to validate the efficacy, methods of preparation, and storage of the remedies. I have written more than a hundred theses and dissertations about the usefulness of homeopathic remedies, in partnership with the Northern Paris Faculty of Medicine (la Faculté de Médecine de Paris Nord), the Paris V Faculty of Pharmacy (la Faculté de Pharmacie de Paris V), and the INSERMs (research facilities) of the Saint-Antoine Hospital in Paris (Dr. William Rostène's department) and of the Percy Hospital at Clamart.

The limits of homeopathy

As with any therapy, homeopathy has its limits. It would be inappropriate to claim that it can cure everything, just as it is inappropriate to claim that allopathy cures everything. We are in the twenty-first century, and it is up to homeopaths to practice a form of homeopathy for the twenty-first century.

With the progress of science and understanding, we should be able to understand and develop our knowledge and to determine the exact limits of homeopathy.

SUCCESS IN SERIOUS ILLNESSES

During the war, some of my teachers, such as Dr. Deloupy, successfully treated serious illnesses such as diphtheria and typhoid.

These days, it is out of the question to treat diphtheria, streptococcus, or serious bacterial pharyngitis in this way. You can treat viral pharyngitis with homeopathy, but a bacterial component necessitates antibiotics, even if you eventually need homeopathy to eliminate the side effects and toxic or detrimental side effects of the medicines.

TREATMENTS COMBINED WITH ALLOPATHY

It is very possible, in the case of cancer, for example, to prescribe chemotherapy or even radiation and homeopathic remedies together to avoid side effects such as hair loss, intense fatigue, nausea, and so on. Homeopathy can, therefore, be very useful in this context, but only alongside allopathic treatment.

CHOOSING THE MOST EFFECTIVE TREATMENT

With a potentially serious illness, it is absolutely essential to follow these two steps:

1. Diagnose the illness (without forgetting the patient and their behavior).
2. Determine if it is possible to use homeopathic treatment. If I had to choose between homeopathy and allopathy, I would always prefer homeopathy, because it has fewer side effects. But when the allopathic therapeutic possibilities are greater, you should not hesitate to use them.

CHAPTER 2

HOMEOPATHIC TREATMENT

How do you treat yourself with homeopathy?

Who can treat themselves with homeopathy?

ANYONE CAN BE TREATED WITH HOMEOPATHY: babies, children, adults, women, men, pregnant women, senior citizens and the elderly, crayfish, cats, dogs, horses, elephants, and even, in certain cases, some plants.

ANIMALS

I have obtained results working with a highly qualified biologist, Amato, who was worried about the crayfish he was breeding. At that time, France, which had previously been an exporter of crayfish, had become an importer, due to a devastating illness that affected the musculature of these animals, preventing them from mating and reproducing.

We carried out an experiment with two separate tanks. In tank A, we put the crayfish in ordinary water; in tank B, we added homeopathic dilutions to the water. We recorded 35 percent fewer deaths in tank B.

I have friends who are specialists in veterinary homeopathy who use homeopathy a great deal, as much for pets as for farm animals or those in captivity.

PLANTS

I have been asked to treat plant pathologies. I shall describe two of them.

To fight mildew at a winery producing organic champagne, we sprayed the vines with a homeopathic solution, and without any other treatment, the harvest was able to proceed normally.

We saved a banana plantation in the Antilles using homeopathic dilutions that enabled the normal development of the bananas with no other treatment.

Other experiments have been carried out on the development of plants by different laboratories; all proved to have a good response to treatment with homeopathic dilutions.

How do you identify your illness?

The first thing to do is to consult a doctor for a medical diagnosis, which is often necessary to know. It may be difficult to differentiate, for example, between the flu and simple asthenia, or between regular sore throat and serious strep throat.

DIAGNOSIS IS INDISPENSABLE

Diagnosis of the illness is absolutely necessary before considering treatment. You should not hesitate to undergo lab tests or X-rays, or consult a specialist.

THE DIFFERENCE BETWEEN THE SYMPTOMS OF AN ILLNESS AND THE HOMEOPATHIC INDICATIONS FOR THE PATIENT

The diagnosis is established by observing the common symptoms of the illness (for the flu: fatigue, muscle pain, high temperature; for Parkinson's: resting tremor and stiffness, walking with small steps, very small handwriting), but to determine the ideal homeopathic treatment, you have to do further research.

In fact, Parkinson's disease could occur subsequent to a traumatic injury (as was the case for Muhammad Ali) or due to industrial poisoning (which was the case for some people who worked in manganese mines), mercury pollution (responsible for a Parkinsonian tremor) or lead (which causes Parkinsonian stiffness), medicines such as neuroleptics, or even in some cases, food (eating too many chickpeas, leading to lathyrism, or too many broad beans, leading to favism, may be at the root of symptoms resembling Parkinson's, which are fortunately reversible once the diet is changed). For each situation, you would prescribe a different remedy. That is because homeopathy is not so interested in the flu as in the person who has the flu, not so much in Parkinson's as in the person with Parkinson's. That is where it is completely different from allopathy. You do not treat pain, but the person who has the pain. It is easy to give a painkiller, but to know how, why, and what conditions the sick person is suffering from, is, in my opinion, one of the main interests of homeopathy: define the person as precisely as possible in order to understand the person better.

That is why the homeopathic practitioner will always be keen to know the patients—their habits and general behavior—as well as possible.

When can you self-medicate? When do you need to consult a practitioner?

You can treat yourself for minor ailments, such as headaches or premenstrual syndrome, without any danger. But it is not so simple to choose the right remedy. Self-medication can come up against two main problems.

First, it can be difficult, even for an expert in homeopathy, to know their own unique remedy. The natural tendency is to choose the remedy according to the symptoms, so they treat the illness rather than the person who is ill. Then it is sometimes tricky to find the right remedy for a pathology—even a common one like the simple cold—for the person who has the cold.

LET'S RESORT TO THE COMPLEX . . .
WITHOUT HAVING COMPLEXES!

For example, Allium cepa is indicated if the person has a runny nose and the wings of the nostrils are irritated. But Euphrasia is better if the eyes are red and irritated; Pulsatilla if the discharge is yellowish and non-irritating; Naphtalinum if the eyes and the nose are irritated and run as if with water; Kali bichromicum if the patient has a yellowish, viscous discharge with crusts and sometimes traces of blood; Mercurius solubilis if the discharge becomes greenish; Nux vomica if the nose is blocked at night and runs during the day; and so on.

Knowing the development of the pathology is very important for choosing the right remedy. In self-medication, if the person knows a lot about homeopathy, they can, perhaps, take many alternating remedies, according to the development of symptoms. But when there is doubt or when you have difficulty finding a pharmacy open and cannot predict the development of the symptoms, it is simpler to use a complex remedy, where there is a combination of Allium cepa, Euphrasia, Belladonna if there is a slight fever, Hydrastis, Kali bichromicum, and Mercurius solubilis. With a combination that contains different remedies for different stages of the pathology, the organism will make its choice of the remedies.

It is, therefore, essential to know the right remedy and the development of the pathology, and you should not hesitate to use good complex remedies.

IF THE SYMPTOMS PERSIST

In any case, you should not take the risk of not noticing a serious illness (for example, a serious infection, depression, a cancerous tumor) by self-medicating too much. If symptoms persist, do not hesitate to consult your doctor or ask for advice from your pharmacist. Normally, a good homeopathic remedy can work in one day (in the case of a slight edema or chill, for example), even within the hour or few minutes following its absorption via the tongue (you allow the remedy to dissolve under the tongue). The active substance is not slowed down by digestive barriers before entering the bloodstream and so can act very rapidly.

WHICH FORM OF TREATMENT SHOULD YOU CHOOSE?

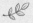

There are three methods of treatment with homeopathic remedies: single remedy (treating the whole person with one remedy), pluralism (polypharmacy, using more than one remedy at a time), and complex homeopathy (treating one person with a number of remedies combined together).

Single remedy

When homeopaths use a single remedy for one subject, the remedy is the one judged to correspond perfectly to the profile of the person. This technique, which some consider to be the flagship of homeopathy, is dependent on the homeopathic doctor alone. For my part, I think it is difficult to find one's specific remedy. You have to be a good homeopath for this method because, in case of error, you leave the patient without treatment, which is damaging to the patient, to the practitioner, and for homeopathy in general.

Pluralism

Pluralists use one remedy for each moment or each stage of the illness.

If the patient develops an ongoing pathology, like rhinitis, the homeopathic doctor will prescribe one or two products, according to the possible developments of the illness, from the symptoms the homeopath is able to observe. The doctor will then be able to rectify the choice of a remedy or the dose by phone. This is the method used by the majority of homeopaths.

Complex prescribing

Homeopaths who use complex remedies combine several remedies in the same bottle to form a combination, which, in this case, is not used according to the behavior of the patient. For rhinitis, for example, it is the remedy for the cold and not the subject who has the cold.

It is also the remedy for the day before the weekend: if the homeopath will not see the patient for several days and is not sure of the development of the illness, the homeopath will prescribe a combination, to be on the safe side.

Is there a good time to take homeopathic remedies?

Finally, people are beginning to take into account the time when the symptoms are most likely to appear, our hormonal output, and the ideal time to take remedies to achieve maximum efficacy.

CHRONOBIOLOGY EXPLAINS ONE ASPECT OF HOMEOPATHIC PRACTICE

Chronobiology has enabled us to understand that the body naturally produces cortisone at about 8 a.m. Therefore, for nearly two hundred years, we have known that asthma symptoms can be aggravated between 1 and 3 a.m. (the time when cortisone is lowest) and then improve at about 8 a.m. Thus, some homeopathic remedies may be chosen according to the aggravation time for the symptoms.

Arsenicum album is thus recommended in the case of symptoms between 1 and 3 a.m., Kalium carbonicum if it is between 2 and 4 a.m., Hyoscyamus niger for a cough that starts as soon as the patient lies down, Drosera for a night cough, Sulphur if the person is awakened at about 5 in the morning by an urgent feeling of diarrhea, Lachesis for morning fatigue, Sepia for fatigue appearing at about 11 in the morning. All these observations collected in the course of homeopathic practice are now, bit by bit, being explained by chronobiology. It is, therefore, important not to forget to choose the right remedy that fits the symptom aggravation or amelioration time.

KNOWING HOW TO OBSERVE IN ORDER TO ANTICIPATE

If you can foresee an aggravation of symptoms at night, you can take the remedy before going to bed. If premenstrual syndrome starts at ovulation, about the fourteenth day of the cycle, with a characteristic migraine, breast tenderness, and abdominal pains that diminish when the period arrives, you would advise taking Folliculinum on the fourteenth day of the cycle.

To research the time when symptoms develop or diminish is good, but it is also necessary to know how to predict, in order to take the appropriate remedy at the right moment.

What form does the homeopathic remedy take?

A homeopathic remedy can take different forms. The most traditional and most often used are pillules, granules, and liquid drops. Each has some advantages and specific benefits.

DRY FORMS

Pillules and globules

Pillules and globules are spherical and differ in size. There are 20 pillules or 200 globules in a gram. These spherical remedies, composed of lactose and sucrose (sugars), are medicated with the homeopathic remedy and have the same name as the substance and dilution.

This is the most effective form of remedy when repeated doses are needed. You will take, for example, 2 pillules 3 times a day at the start of treatment, then space out the doses once symptoms improve. You completely stop treatment when symptoms disappear.

Granules

Granules are provided in doses and are limited to one single dose, whether to remove a physical or psychological obstacle, or in case of chronic pathology.

The remedy may, then, be taken weekly, biweekly, monthly, or even annually, according to the pathologies concerned.

For example, in case of hematoma or bruising caused by physical trauma, you can take a dose of Arnica montana 9 CH. In case of anxiety or panic due to a psychological shock such as a car accident, you would advise a dose of the same remedy, but in 15 CH.

If an anxious person has to pass an exam, you would prescribe a dose of Gelsemium in 9 CH.

Powders

Powders are used for insoluble active substances in low dilutions and are mixed with lactose. Calcarea carbonica, for example, will be used in 8 DH to treat and strengthen bones.

Tablets

Tablets are similar powders, but their compact form is often more convenient. They are manufactured by compressing homeopathic powder or by medicating a blank tablet with tincture. They are also labeled with the name of the substance and its dilution: for example, Nux vomica 5 CH in tablet form.

Their psychological value is obvious because they resemble a standard allopathic remedy. However, it is necessary to avoid swallowing them whole; rather, they should be sucked or allowed to dissolve under the tongue (like granules or pillules), in order for them to penetrate directly into the circulatory system and avoid traveling first through the digestive system, which will slow the action of medicines and diminish the effect.

LIQUID FORMS

These are mainly used as complex remedies. For example, for good liver drainage, you would choose a complex of Taraxacum (for the median lobe), Chelidonium majus (for the right lobes), and Carduus marianus (for the left lobe). The combination of these three remedies will drain the whole liver.

Mother tincture

The action of the mother tincture is phytotherapeutic. For example, Orthosiphon is a diuretic; Fucus vesiculosus is a diuretic and thyroid stimulant and is used during weight loss programs.

Liquid remedies in vials

Liquid remedies in vials are not of greater therapeutic benefit than other forms of remedies, but they have the advantage of simplifying treatment. To use them, you would take 1 vial or 40 drops a day in an appropriate dilution. This form is frequently used in lithotherapy (Versailles limestone 8 DH, for example).

AND ALSO . . .

Creams and ointments

These are applied to the skin for local treatment, or when a patient is too sensitive to the homeopathic remedy for it to be taken internally. Hahnemann used them frequently.

Calendula cream would be advised for its antiseptic properties. Massage with Bryonia will soothe pains that are better with pressure and rest.

Suppositories and ovules

These are used for local treatment. Aesculus hippocastanum suppositories would, therefore, be suggested in the treatment of hemorrhoids, or Hydrastis calendula in the case of benign vaginal irritation.

Which dilution should you choose?

There is a simple prescription for dilutions of remedies, depending on the nature of the symptoms:

- For local symptoms, choose low dilutions (4–5 CH).

- For general symptoms, choose moderate strength dilutions (7–9 CH).

- For mental/emotional symptoms or chronic illnesses, choose high dilutions (15–30 CH).

For example, Arsenicum album may be used at 5 CH to treat local eczema on the pinna of the ear if there is also a burning sensation and the pain improves with heat (it is a local symptom). You would prescribe a dilution of 9 CH of this same remedy in the case of food poisoning with nausea, diarrhea, and burning abdominal pains that are helped by heat (these are general symptoms). Finally, an anxious, agitated asthmatic having attacks at 1 and 3 a.m. would also be treated with Arsenicum album, but in the 15 CH potency (because it is more a matter of mental/emotional symptoms).

How do you choose the dose for homeopathic remedies?

We are not going to talk about the quantity of medicines in relation to weight or age, as you might in allopathy. The way that the remedy works is different, and honestly, whether you take one, two, or three pillules, it comes to exactly the same thing. We are not talking quantitatively, but qualitatively, and you should be able to treat a mouse or an elephant, a baby or an adult, with the same dilution and the same dose of the remedy. However, it would always be advisable, as a precaution, to take several pillules in one dose. You cannot ignore the risk that during the process of manufacturing of the remedies, one or two pillules may not have been medicated. When you process 500 kilograms of pillules, it is possible, even if the techniques are well validated, that some pillules "escape" the active substance. It is, therefore, preferable to take at least 2 or 3 pillules, to be certain of having at least one that is effective.

How do you take homeopathic remedies?

PILLULES, GRANULES, OR DROPS: WHICH FORM OF REMEDY SHOULD YOU CHOOSE?

For an adult, I always advise taking the remedy in the form of drops, because you can shake it, which reactivates the solution and makes it possible to obtain a new remedy with a different potency each time. But this form is sometimes less practical in the circumstances of modern daily life (at the office, on public transportation), and it is often simpler to take a small tube of pillules or a single dose with you, rather than a bottle that could break. You can always alternate the form of remedy you take: the formula drops at home, and pillules elsewhere.

KNOWING HOW TO TRANSLATE DOSES

You can take your medication using two different forms of the same remedy—the same product, in the same dilution:

5–8 pillules = 1 dose

2–3 pillules = 5–6 drops

IS IT TRUE THAT YOU SHOULD NOT
TOUCH PILLULES WITH YOUR FINGERS?

Previously, homeopathic remedies were predominantly manu-factured in very compact pillules. When they were medicated with the active substance, it remained on the surface, and due to the infinitesimal dilution, even slight perspiration or damp-ness on the fingers would risk dissolving the active principle, thus rendering the remedy ineffective.

Today, thanks to the composition of pillules (lactose and sucrose) and new manufacturing techniques, the active prin-ciple passes, by absorption and capillary action, to the interior of the support substance.

So you can, now, touch them without altering their efficacy. But for hygienic reasons, if you have been in contact with an essential oil, it is still preferable to take the remedy using the dosing cap provided for this purpose.

IS IT TRUE THAT YOU SHOULD NOT SWALLOW THEM
LIKE A STANDARD PILL?

The ideal way that the pillule or the homeopathic dose is absorbed is via the tongue. The remedy is allowed to dissolve under the tongue, which takes a few minutes. In this way, the active substance passes directly into the bloodstream without being slowed down by digestive barriers, and thus acts more effectively and quickly.

If the homeopathic remedy is intended for a baby or an animal, you need to use other means of administration.

HOW DO YOU GIVE HOMEOPATHIC REMEDIES TO A BABY OR AN ANIMAL?

For a baby, I prefer to give the homeopathic remedy in the form of drops (shake the bottle well before giving a remedy to a child) that do not contain alcohol, despite the inconvenience that the remedy will keep for only a short time. Keep the remedy in the refrigerator, use it in a few days, and do not hesitate to discard it after 5 or 6 days. You could also dissolve pillules in milk. Pillules, being made of lactose and sucrose, dissolve in milk (or in water) very well. A baby bottle is a very good conduit. By feeding on it, the baby will quickly absorb the remedy via the tongue.

It is easy to slip a pillule into pet food or into an apple that you give a horse to munch.

IS IT TRUE THAT YOU SHOULD NOT TAKE HOMEOPATHIC REMEDIES DURING OR AFTER A MEAL?

Because the ideal method of absorption is via the tongue, it is preferable to take the homeopathic remedy at least 30 minutes before a meal or 1 hour afterward.

When you eat, the tongue is already absorbing food and drink, so the remedy risks being assimilated more slowly. As a general rule, it is preferable to take homeopathic remedies and meals at different times.

IS IT TRUE THAT SOME PRODUCTS ADVERSELY AFFECT THE EFFICACY OF HOMEOPATHY?

There can be incompatibilities. Avoid chamomile, which is a general antidote to any homeopathic product, and essential oils. Never open a bottle of essential oil next to a homeopathic remedy: it could inhibit its action. The remedy comes in infinitesimal dilution, while the essential oils are very concentrated and have a very powerful effect. It is for this reason that you should never manufacture homeopathic products and products based on essential oils on the same premises.

It is generally preferable to keep stimulants, such as coffee or mint, away from remedies. They cause a slight constriction of the taste buds, which slows down the absorption of the active substance. But you do not have to completely avoid mint; just take your remedy well before or after you brush your teeth, eat a mentholated sweet, or drink mint tea.

IT IS TRUE THAT THE REMEDY IS NO LONGER ACTIVE AFTER THE SELL-BY DATE?

- Pillules or granules may be used after the sell-by date, as can drops in liquid potency and in medicating potency.

- Mother tinctures should not be used after the sell-by date because there can be sedimentation of the active substance or evaporation of the solvent.

- In any case, you should keep homeopathic remedies away from light, extremes of temperature, and humidity.

How long should treatment be continued?

Duration of treatment depends on the type of pathology.

LOCAL SYMPTOMS, ACUTE PATHOLOGY

If the symptoms are local or the pathology acute (for example, a cold, asthma attack, or eczema flare-up), you take the remedy in low dilution (4–5 CH), 4 to 5 times a day, until the symptoms subside.

When the person feels better, space out the doses, and then stop them completely when the symptoms disappear. Continuation of treatment risks causing a proving—a pathology or symptoms not triggered by the illness but by repeated and excessive doses of the same remedy. Consider the case of a person who has been coughing for more than a month. Treated with Drosera, they continue their treatment when the symptoms begin to subside. They are still coughing today, but the cough is now caused by the remedy. It would be enough to stop taking it for their symptoms to disappear completely.

Ailments completely different from the initial pathology may also appear. I have seen a case of a person who was treated with Sepia for repeated cystitis. Over a period of time, the remedy caused slight depression, from which the person, fortunately, recovered simply by stopping the remedy.

GENERAL SYMPTOMS

In the case of more general treatment (such as tiredness or pregnancy), use average-strength doses (7–9 CH), take the remedies regularly and repeatedly (2 to 3 times a day), and stop when the person feels better.

CHRONIC OR MENTAL/EMOTIONAL SYMPTOMS

In case of chronic pathology (such as rheumatism) or mental/emotional problems, choose very high dilutions (15–30 CH) and administer regularly in doses taken at regular intervals: for example, once a week or once a month.

IF SYMPTOMS PERSIST

In the case of acute pathology, such as a cold, if the symptoms persist for longer than 2–3 days without improving, this may be because:

- You have chosen the wrong remedy, and it is ineffective for treating your symptoms. Stop taking it and change it with the help, where necessary, of a doctor or homeopathic pharmacist.

- You have taken your remedy for too long; stop taking it.

- You are missing the diagnosis of a more serious illness; you need to see a doctor.

CHAPTER 3

SELECTING REMEDIES: WHICH ONE FOR WHICH SYMPTOM?

Identify your symptoms and treat them.

Where is the problem?

LOCATE YOUR SYMPTOM.

THE HEAD

HEAD	
Injury/swelling	Migraine
Headache	
EYES	
Cataracts	Stye
Conjunctivitis	Dryness of the eyes
Ocular fatigue	Sensitivity to light
Black eye	Twitching eyelids

NOSE

Coryza, nasal discharge	Polyps
Sneezing	Rhinitis, cold
Blocked nose	Bleeding sinusitis

EARS

Buzzing/ringing in the ears (tinnitus)	Otitis

MOUTH

Abscess	Dry lips, chapped lips
Mouth ulcers	Bad breath
Cold sores	Teething
Cavities	Bleeding gums
Pain—teeth	Sensitivity of teeth to heat or cold
Gingivitis	

THROAT

Sore throat	Laryngitis, pharyngitis
Aphonia	Strep throat
Hoarseness	Problems with deglutition (swallowing)
Tonsillitis	
Cough, tracheitis	

NECK

Whiplash	Stiffness, torticollis
Pain—neck	

FACE

Acne	Blemishes
Eczema	Tics
Diffuse redness	

HAIR

Greasy hair

Dull, brittle hair

Hair falling out

Dandruff

THORAX

Intercostal pain

Intercostal neuralgia (shingles)

HEART

Palpitations

LUNGS, RESPIRATION

Asthma

Bronchitis

Bronchiolitis

Hiccups

Snoring

CHEST

Pain—breast

Engorgement after giving birth

ABDOMEN

DIGESTIVE ORGANS

Flatulence (eructations, burps), bloating

Calculi

Burning sensation—stomach

Constipation

Colic

Diarrhea

Indigestion—liver problems

Fissure, anal fistula

Stomach pain

Flatulence, gas

Hangover

Gastroenteritis

Food poisoning

Fecal incontinence

Drunkenness

Acid reflux, regurgitations

Nausea, vomiting

Stomach ulcers

Gastritis

ABDOMEN (continued)

URINARY ORGANS

Kidney stones

Cystitis, urinary tract infection

Incontinence, bedwetting (enuresis)

GENITAL ORGANS

Premature ejaculation

Fibroma

Genital herpes

Impotence

Menstruation

Menopause

Mycosis

Vaginal discharge

Prostate (problems with)

BACK

Pain

Low back pain

Back pain

Sciatica

Scoliosis

Trauma and shock

LIMBS

Osteoarthritis

Cellulite

Sprains

Muscle pain

Cramps

Torn muscle

Pain—joints

Pain—limbs

Pain—muscle

Pain—tendons

Pulled muscle

Strains

Fractures

Luxation

Tendonitis

HANDS AND FEET

Dermatitis (hands and feet)

Swelling of fingers

Clammy hands

Brittle, double, or stained nails

Paronychia

Warts around the nails

Foot sweat

HOMEOPATHY

SKELETAL SYSTEM

Pain—bones

Fractures

Osteoporosis

CIRCULATORY SYSTEM

Varicose eczema

Circulation problems

Hemorrhoids

Tired, heavy legs

Phlebitis

Weakening of the veins

Venous ulcers

Varicose veins

SKIN

Abscess, cyst

Acne

Bruise, hematoma

Injury/swelling

Cold sores

Burns

Cellulite

Scarring

Blow, trauma

Sunburn

Cut

Fissure

Irritation, itching

Abrasion

Eczema

Erythema of the buttocks—
    diaper rash in babies

Boil

Herpes

Chapped skin

Panaritium

Jaundice, yellow skin

Insect bite/sting

Dry skin

Blemishes

Diffuse redness

Urticaria

Excessive perspiration

Herpes zoster (shingles)

Warts

MENTAL/EMOTIONAL

Despondency

Anguish, anxiety

Postpartum depression

Excessive appetite

Emotional shock

Emotional intensity

MENTAL/EMOTIONAL (continued)

Excitability

Mental and emotional
  hypersensitivity

Insomnia

Jealousy

Logorrhea (tendency to talk
  continuously)

Memory problems

Nervousness, stress

Fear, stage fright

Panic

Tics

GENERAL STATE

Alcoholism

Allergies

Emaciation, weight loss

Anemia

Sore throat

Appetite

Asthenia, apathy

Asthma

Bronchiolitis

Bronchitis

Blow

Indigestion, liver problems

Diabetes

Weakness, fatigue, burnout

Brain fatigue

Gastroenteritis

Fever

Flu

Gout

Hyperactivity

Hepatitis

Staphylococcus infection

Hypertension

Altitude sickness

Sunstroke

Obesity

Motion sickness

Parkinson's

Surgical operation

Stunted growth

Rickets

Measles

Educational underachievement

Spasms

Rubella

Smoking

Spasmophilia (latent tetany)

Tremor

Traumatization and shock

Chicken pox

Vaccination and vaccination
  damage

Worms

Vertigo

Aging

Birth	Constipation
Acidity	Nausea
Breastfeeding	Nervousness, stress
Postpartum depression	Water retention
Circulation	

List of symptoms and their treatment

Remember: with all homeopathic treatment, take the remedy less often when you feel better and stop taking it as soon as the symptoms cease. The following dosage, therefore, is applicable to symptoms at the initial stage of treatment. It deliberately does not include details of duration. It is up to you to adjust it according to your response to treatment.

DESPONDENCY

See: Apathy, asthenia, dejection, page 73; Weakness, fatigue, burnout, page 161.

ABSCESS, BOIL, PANARITIUM

Skin infection with concentration of pus. In the case of a boil, staphylococcus is often an issue.

To start, you will just see a red, painful patch with a white head that may be more or less yellowish in the middle, and then the pus accumulates. The pain may be very acute; you are sensitive to the slightest touch.

INDICATIONS	TREATMENT
The abscess is red, hot, even burning, and painful	Belladonna 5 CH 2 pillules 3 times a day
The abscess is ready to burst; use what is called the homeopathic lancet	Myristica 5 CH 2 pillules 3 times a day
The abscess begins to discharge	*To promote discharge* Hepar sulphur 5 CH 2 pillules 3 times a day *combined with* Pyrogenium 9 CH 2 pillules 3 times a day
The pus has discharged	*To regulate or stop discharge* Hepar sulphur 9 CH 2 pillules 3 times a day *then* Hepar sulphur 15 CH 2 pillules 3 times a day
The area of the abscess is purplish, the pain is acute, and you have a fever	*While waiting to see the doctor or in combination with antibiotics* Tarentula cubensis 5 CH 2 pillules 3 times a day *combined with* Pyrogenium 9 CH 2 pillules 3 times a day
These infections recur in a chronic manner and you are sensitive to cold	Silicea 5 CH 2 pillules 3 times a day *combined with* Pyrogenium 9 CH 2 pillules 3 times a day

INDICATIONS	TREATMENT
When there is a boil	*Add, in all cases* Staphylococcinum 5 CH 2 pillules 3 times a day
In case of surgical operation, if the abscess has been opened with a pointed object	*Add* Hypericum perforatum 5 CH 2 pillules 3 times a day
In case of surgical operation, if the abscess has been opened with a cutting object such as a lancet	*Add* Staphysagria 5 CH 2 pillules 3 times a day
In all cases	*Local application of* Calendula cream *or* Calendula mother tincture *or* Echinacea mother tincture *or* Mimosa tenuiflora mother tincture
There is a dental abscess	*Mouthwash with the combination* Calendula officinalis mother tincture Echinacea purpurea mother tincture Phytolacca mother tincture 25 to 30 drops diluted in a half glass of tepid water 2 to 3 times a day (as needed) Bottle of 30 ml prepared by your pharmacist

Do not keep touching an abscess. Do not try to compress it, pierce it, or discharge the pus manually. An urgent medical consultation is needed if:

- It is located on the face or close to the genital organs.

- It does not heal or it causes a flare-up of boils; antibiotics can sometimes be essential.

- There is a dental abscess.

- You have a fever.

- It is a recurrent abscess, which may indicate a predisposition to diabetes.

BIRTH

See: Pregnancy, page 181.

ACNE

The "pimples" of puberty, resulting from a burst of hormones that occurs to ensure the development of sexual attributes. The sebaceous glands, which normally provide a protective sebum for the skin, tend to become erratic. This imbalance induces the development of comedones—small blackheads—and of small, closed cysts on the forehead, the chin, and sometimes all over the face. When they become inflamed, this can lead to pustules, which sometimes proliferate.

INDICATIONS	TREATMENT
The acne is situated around the lips, on dry lips	Natrum muriaticum 5 CH 2 pillules 3 times a day
The acne is situated on the forehead and on the back	Sulphur iodatum 5 CH 2 pillules 3 times a day
It is a case of intractable acne that discharges pus and leaves scars	Kalium bromatum 5 CH 2 pillules 3 times a day
The skin is greasy and you feel tired	Selenium 5 CH 2 pillules 3 times a day
The skin is unhealthy, you often feel too hot, and water and heat increase the irritation	Sulfur 5 CH 2 pillules 3 times a day
The acne is due to a staphylococcus	Staphylococcinum 5 CH 2 pillules 3 times a day *combined with* Pyrogenium 9 CH 2 pillules 3 times a day
The acne is aggravated before menstruation and diminishes when it arrives and the pus is discharged	*With the agreement of your homeopathic doctor* Folliculinum 9 CH 1 dose on the 14th day of the cycle *To accelerate elimination* Hepar sulphur 5 CH 2 pillules 3 times a day *combined with* Pyrogenium 9 CH 2 pillules 3 times a day

Do not squeeze, burst, or keep touching! Self-image is important, especially in adolescence, and seeing oneself "disfigured" is difficult to tolerate, but it will not help to keep touching your spots: completely the opposite! You will only create additional redness and irritation; moreover, the toxins and microbes could then enter the bloodstream.

Forget about food that is fatty (sausages, French fries, and the like). Eat a healthy diet, drink a lot of liquids, and tell yourself that puberty is an indispensable stage in the creation of a human being, and it only happens once.

TINNITUS

See: Buzzing and ringing in the ear (Tinnitus), page 92.

FLATULENCE (ERUCTATIONS, BURPS), BLOATING

Burps and expulsion of air and gas (flatulence) in general are linked to swelling of the abdomen (bloating) and to digestive problems.

INDICATIONS	TREATMENT
The bloating is below the navel; it appears from the beginning of a meal and/or between 4:00 and 8:00 p.m.	Lycopodium 5 CH 2 pillules 3 times a day
The bloating is above the navel	Carbo vegetabilis 5 CH 2 pillules 3 times a day

INDICATIONS	TREATMENT
The bloating is both above and below the navel	China rubra 5 CH (*Cinchona officinalis*) 2 pillules 3 times a day
You suffer from increasing bloating with a feeling of breathlessness in the chest	Asafoetida 5 CH 2 pillules 3 times a day
Your bloating is accompanied by copious, liquid, intense diarrhea	Podophyllum peltatum 5 CH 2 pillules 3 times a day
Your bloating is accompanied by liver problems and constipation	Raphanus sativus 5 CH 2 pillules 3 times a day
Your flatulence, which is better when sitting, makes you weak	Kalium carbonicum 5 CH 2 pillules 3 times a day

ADVICE

- Eat slowly and chew well when eating meals.

- Eat in a calm atmosphere and at regular times.

- Avoid activities in which you could swallow air when not eating meals (for example, chewing gum).

- Avoid all foods that ferment easily (for example, cabbage, sauerkraut, beans) and carbonated beverages.

- Make use of herbs. Cumin is frequently used in Mediterranean cooking to flavor beans, and it helps digest them. It also decreases the formation of gas, as does green aniseed.

ALCOHOLISM

Chronic abuse of alcohol with dependency. Alcoholism is very difficult to treat with homeopathy, but you can help to influence the behavior of the person who is ill.

INDICATIONS	TREATMENT
You notice an aggravation of your condition and sleepiness after meals, or you wish to prevent a possible hangover	Nux vomica 5 CH 2 pillules 30 minutes before the meal
Your alcoholism is due to your social or professional life	Nux vomica 5 CH 2 pillules 30 minutes before the meal
Your alcoholism is accompanied by extreme talkativeness; your face is red, even purplish; and you dislike having anything tight round your neck (necklace, tie, turtleneck)	Lachesis 9 CH 2 pillules 3 times a day
The alcoholism is accompanied by nervous tics	Agaricus muscarius 5 CH 2 pillules 3 times a day
The alcoholism is well established	Ethylicum 7 CH 2 pillules 3 times a day *Repeat the dose every time you want a drink*

INDICATIONS	TREATMENT
The alcoholism has been well established for a long time and is accompanied by cirrhosis, acid reflux, and tremors	Sulphuricum acidum 5 CH 2 pillules 3 times a day

ADVICE

Alcoholism is a chronic condition, which can give rise to other, equally serious illnesses (cirrhosis of the liver, cancer, and so on). The patient affected needs help. It is essential to consult a doctor and/or a psychologist.

BREASTFEEDING

This is not an illness, but feeding a baby may be more difficult than you had expected (lack of milk or breast engorgement) and cause ailments (such as cracked nipples).

INDICATIONS	TREATMENT
WHEN THE MILK COMES IN	
To help the milk come in	Agnus castus 5 CH 2 pillules 3 times a day
To improve breastfeeding and help the milk come in	Pulsatilla 9 CH 2 pillules 3 times a day
To promote the production of milk	Baryta carbonicum 9 CH 2 pillules 3 times a day
To promote breastfeeding	Ricinus communis 5 CH (Castor oil) 2 pillules 3 times a day

INDICATIONS	TREATMENT
BREAST ENGORGEMENT	
The breasts are swollen, red, and painful	Belladonna 5 CH 2 pillules 3 times a day
The breasts are hard, heavy, and painful	Bryonia 5 CH 2 pillules 3 times a day
CRACKED NIPPLES	
Cracks have formed	Graphites 5 CH 2 pillules 3 times a day
WEANING	
To dry up the milk secretion	*For 3 to 4 days* Ricinus communis 15 CH 2 pillules 3 times a day *combined with* Pulsatilla 5 CH 2 pillules 3 times a day

ADVICE

A lot of water, rest, and love: that is generally all a mother needs to succeed at breastfeeding. But sometimes just the baby being in the wrong position while feeding or the mother's lack of self-confidence can prevent the process from going smoothly. Do not remain isolated with your problem: speak about it to people around you, to midwives, to breastfeeding organizations, to your mother, your friends. There is nothing like the experience of others to rediscover these natural movements that ensure that the baby has an irreplaceable form of nourishment at the earliest stage of life and that the mother has moments of unforgettable tenderness and bonding with the baby.

To dry up the production of milk at the end of breast-feeding, drink a purgative lemonade or use a laxative or a purgative to help you: it's very effective! But be careful when you do this to make sure that you have completely stopped breast-feeding your baby, who would otherwise risk ingesting these substances.

ALLERGIES

Extreme reactions to substances called allergens, of which there are a great many: house dust, dust mites, insect stings, animal hair, pollen, food (shellfish, milk, peanuts, soy), medicines, pollution, pesticides, heavy metals, dyes, makeup, soap, clothing fibers, climate (humidity, cold), sun.

Allergies can cause asthma, edema, coughs, nasal discharge, inflammations, eczema, and urticaria.

INDICATIONS	TREATMENT
ENT ALLERGIES	
The eyes water and are irritated	Histaminum 5 CH 2 pillules 3 times a day *combined with* Euphrasia 5 CH 2 pillules 3 times a day
The allergy causes sneezing fits	Histaminum 5 CH 2 pillules 3 times a day, or more in case of an acute attack *combined with* Sabadilla 5 CH 2 pillules 3 times a day

INDICATIONS	TREATMENT
The wings of the nostrils are irritated	Histaminum 5 CH 2 pillules 3 times a day *combined with* Allium cepa 5 CH 2 pillules 3 times a day
RESPIRATORY ALLERGIES	
The allergy causes a cough	Lung histamine 5 CH 2 pillules 3 times a day *or* Lung histamine 9 CH 1 dose *combined with* a homeopathic cough remedy of choice, according to the cough *(See: Complex remedies, page 320)*
The bronchi are clogged up; you have difficulty expectorating, but you feel better when you can	Antimonium tartaricum 5 CH 2 pillules 3 times a day
The allergy causes an asthma attack	Ethyl sulfur dichloratum 5 CH 2 pillules 3 to 4 times a day *combined with* Lung histamine 5 CH 2 pillules 3 times a day *(See also: Asthma, page 85)*
It is an allergy to pollens, grasses, trees, and the like	Pollen 5 CH 2 pillules 3 times a day

INDICATIONS	TREATMENT
SKIN ALLERGIES	
In the case of an allergy to the sun: the skin is red, hot, painful, and it burns	Belladonna 5 CH 2 pillules 3 times a day
In the case of an allergy to the sun: it causes a rose-colored edema (like an insect sting) that is better with coolness, even cold (application of ice)	Apis mellifica 5 CH 2 pillules 3 times a day
In the case of an allergy to the sun that produces large blisters	Cantharis 5 CH 2 pillules 3 times a day
In the case of an allergy to the sun in the form of burns and ulcerations	Muriaticum acidum 5 CH 2 pillules 3 times a day
The allergy is due to contact (for example, with dye, makeup, metal), or a food, medicine, or vaccine	Histaminum 5 CH 2 pillules 3 times a day *combined with* Isotherapic of the allergenic substance 5 CH 2 pillules 3 times a day *then* Isotherapic of the allergenic substance 7 CH 2 pillules 3 times a day *(see the advice below)*
The allergy is accompanied by urticaria	Urtica urens 5 CH 2 pillules 3 times a day

INDICATIONS	TREATMENT
IN ALL CASES	
It is a long-standing allergy	The same indications, but increase the potencies (dilutions) to 9 CH, even 15 CH for very long-standing allergies

ADVICE

Where possible, avoid substances you know you are allergic to. In the case of a serious allergy or one that is really disabling, desensitization may also be a useful procedure.

In all cases, if you know the cause of your symptoms, iso-therapy with the substance responsible can be prescribed for you: if you are allergic to house dust or to a particular pollen, give your pharmacist a sample of this dust or this pollen to provide the raw material for the manufacture of the remedy, which you will take for 4 weeks:

- The first week, 5 CH (2 pillules 3 times a day).

- The second week, 7 CH (2 pillules 3 times a day).

- The third week, 9 CH (2 pillules 3 times a day).

- The fourth week, 15 CH (2 pillules 3 times a day).

ISOTHERAPY

An isotherapic remedy is one manufactured from the substance that makes you ill. All you need to do is to take a little of this substance, whatever it may be, to a pharmacy. They will send it to a laboratory that will then be able to manufacture your personalized remedy.

WEIGHT LOSS

Sudden or continued weight loss. Weight loss is often associated with diet but may also be the symptom of a health condition, especially when you still have a good appetite.

INDICATIONS	TREATMENT
For an adolescent who grows up too fast and gets tired too easily, even if they have a lot of energy initially	Natrum muriaticum 5 CH 2 pillules 3 times a day *combined with* Phosphorus 9 CH 1 dose a week *and with* Kalium phosphoricum 5 CH 2 pillules 3 times a day
If, additionally, this adolescent is nervous	*Add to the preceding remedies* Silicea 5 CH 2 pillules 3 times a day
You lose weight without losing appetite, you burn everything up, you are always hot (perhaps you have thyroid problems), and you are agitated	*To regulate thyroid action* Iodum 9 CH 1 dose a week *or* Thyroid 9 CH 1 dose a week *To slow down thyroid action* Iodum 15 CH 1 dose a week *or* Thyroid 15 CH 1 dose a week

INDICATIONS	TREATMENT
Your appetite has not diminished, but you are losing weight, particularly in the upper body, and you are becoming apathetic and nervous	Natrum muriaticum 5 CH 2 pillules 3 times a day *combined with* Silicea 9 CH 1 dose twice a week
You are becoming weak, thin, and nervous; your resistance to infections is diminishing	Tuberculinum aviaire 9 CH 2 pillules 3 times a day

See also: Appetite (lack of), page 81.

ADVICE

In case of prolonged and unexplained weight loss, you have to consider possible thyroid problems, for which it would be better to entrust treatment to a doctor. A diagnosis may prove essential.

ANEMIA

Lowering of the level of red cells in the blood. You feel weak and very tired.

Homeopathy can only treat benign anemia, the consequence of an illness.

INDICATIONS	TREATMENT
The anemia occurs after an eruptive illness (measles, chicken pox, and the like)	China rubra 5 CH (*Cinchona officinalis*) 2 pillules 3 times a day
The anemia occurs after an inflammatory illness	Ferrum phosphoricum 5 CH 2 pillules 3 times a day

INDICATIONS	TREATMENT
The anemia occurs after a hemorrhage (loss of blood)	Phosphorus 9 CH 1 dose *combined with* China rubra 5 CH (*Cinchona officinalis*) 1 pillule 3 times a day

ADVICE

If anemia continues, you should always obtain medical advice. It can be masking another, more serious illness, and sometimes a transfusion could be necessary. In all cases, a blood count and a precise diagnosis are essential and vitally important.

For benign anemias, a diet rich in iron could help the system, on condition that the iron is correctly assimilated. To help with this, consider using Ferrum phosphoricum in Schuessler Tissue Salts 6 DH, at a rate of 2 tablets 3 times a day.

SORE THROAT, TONSILLITIS, THROAT PAIN, PHARYNGITIS

Painful condition of the throat and tonsils, sometimes of viral origin. You have a fever and difficulty swallowing. It is necessary to distinguish between a sore throat with redness and one with white patches.

INDICATIONS	TREATMENT
SORE THROAT WITH REDNESS	
Your throat looks red; you have difficulty swallowing and a high temperature	Belladonna 5 CH 2 pillules 3 times a day

INDICATIONS	TREATMENT
Your throat looks red and your mouth is dry; you have difficulty swallowing, a high temperature, difficulties with salivation, great thirst, dilated pupils. You are very sensitive to light	Belladonna 9 CH 2 pillules 3 times a day
Your tonsils are red and look striated, with scarlet streaks	Phytolacca 5 CH 2 pillules 3 times a day
The tonsils are hard and swollen, especially in a slightly plump and placid child	Baryta carbonicum 5 CH 2 pillules 3 times a day
The sore throat appears after exposure to damp cold	Dulcamara 5 CH 2 pillules 3 times a day
There is slight edema in the area of the neck; you have difficulty in swallowing but you are not thirsty and feel better if ice is applied	Apis mellifica 5 CH 2 pillules 3 times a day *or* Apis mellifica 9 CH 1 dose
A "splinter-like" pain deep in the throat, increased by your hectic lifestyle, makes you cough	Argentum nitricum 5 CH 2 pillules 3 times a day
You have a burning pain, as if you had pepper in your throat	Capsicum annuum 5 CH 2 pillules 3 times a day

INDICATIONS	TREATMENT
You have a pain in a particular spot, which does not extend outward	Kalium bichromicum 5 CH 2 pillules 3 times a day
SORE THROAT WITH WHITENESS	
You salivate profusely; your tongue is white; you have bad breath and chills	Mercurius solubilis 9 CH 2 pillules 3 times a day
The sore throat is right-sided	Mercurius proto-iodatus 5 CH 2 pillules 3 times a day
You have repeated right-sided sore throats and liver problems	Mercurius proto-iodatus 5 CH 2 pillules 3 times a day *combined with* Lycopodium 5 CH 2 pillules 3 times a day
The sore throat is left-sided	Mercurius bi-iodatus 5 CH 2 pillules 3 times a day
You have repeated left-sided sore throats and bruising that appears at random; you talk a great deal	Mercurius bi-iodatus 5 CH 2 pillules 3 times a day *combined with* Lachesis 9 CH 2 pillules 3 times a day
There are small ulcerations in the throat	Mercurius corrosivus 5 CH 2 pillules 3 times a day
There is a veil-like membrane on the palate, and the tonsils are white	*While waiting to consult a doctor* Mercurius cyanatus 5 CH 2 pillules every hour

INDICATIONS	TREATMENT
	IN ALL CASES
As a mouthwash	Phytolacca mother tincture
	and
	Calendula mother tincture
	10 drops of each in a glass of water

See also: Laryngitis, page 207; Hoarseness, aphonia, page 153.

ADVICE

If the homeopathic treatment does not take effect within 2 or 3 days, you should consult a doctor who will give an accurate diagnosis. Be aware, however, that antibiotics, often given to cure sore throats, are totally ineffective in the case of illnesses of viral origin. But if antibiotics are essential, use them with the homeopathic remedies cited above, which will enable you to tolerate them better.

ANGUISH

Extreme anxiety, which causes demonstrable signs of fear. You have palpitations, difficulty in breathing, tension in the throat, and stomach cramps. You feel mentally and emotionally inhibited and unable to react.

These symptoms may appear before the start of an event that you are anticipating or in a situation that you dread. At their most severe, they are capable of disturbing your ability to adapt and can ruin your daily life.

INDICATIONS	TREATMENT
You are agitated, you have the sensation of having a ball in the throat, your anxiety is diminished by being distracted, and it causes you paradoxical reactions (you can swallow sauerkraut in the company of someone you like, but you are incapable of eating yogurt in the company of someone you don't like, for example)	Ignatia amara 5 CH 2 pillules 3 times a day
The anxiety comes on before an oral exam; it is stage fright that inhibits you: you cannot get a word out, you have the feeling that your legs have been cut off	Gelsemium 9 CH 2 pillules the day before the exam 2 pillules 30 minutes before the exam 2 pillules during the exam
The anxiety is subsequent to an accident	Arnica montana 15 CH 2 pillules 3 times a day
The anxiety is triggered by a fever; you are not hungry; you are exhausted and trembling	Gelsemium 9 CH 2 pillules 3 times a day

INDICATIONS	TREATMENT
You are agitated, subject to waking in the night; you are becoming obsessive; you have morbid ideas	Arsenicum album 9 CH 2 pillules 3 times a day *or if mental/emotional problems are very important* Arsenicum album 15 CH 2 pillules 3 times a day
You are very agitated, suffer from vertigo, and would like to have completed everything before starting anything	Argentum nitricum 9 CH 2 pillules 3 times a day *or if mental/emotional problems are very important* Argentum nitricum 15 CH 2 pillules 3 times a day
The anxiety leads to depression and causes you to isolate yourself	Sepia 15 CH 2 pillules 3 times a day
The anxiety is accompanied by slight paranoia or jealousy and you talk without stopping	Lachesis 15 CH 2 pillules 3 times a day
The anxiety is accompanied by loss of memory and you feel better when you eat, which means that you graze all the time	Anacardium orientale 9 CH 2 pillules 3 times a day

ADVICE

When you have a temporary attack of anxiety, breathe! Respiratory exercises (deep inhalations and then complete exhalations) can help to overcome difficulties, regain a peaceful state of mind, and step back from the situation triggering the anxiety. But in case of serious anxiety or anguish accompanied by suicidal or depressive ideas, it is better to make an emergency appointment with a psychologist or a psychiatrist to avoid the risk of a crisis.

ANXIETY

See: Anguish, page 70.

APATHY, ASTHENIA, DEJECTION

Physical or mental/emotional debility, with absence of reaction and of energy. You become indifferent to everything, with neither desire nor emotion. The apathy could be physical or mental/emotional.

INDICATIONS	TREATMENT
You have been worn out since the start of the day; you are sleepy and almost lifeless, physically and mentally/emotionally slow; you are putting on weight and becoming more and more unadventurous	*To treat the attack* Baryta carbonicum 5 CH 2 pillules 3 times a day *then, when the tube is finished* Baryta carbonicum 9 CH 1 dose a week for 1 month *then* Baryta carbonicum 15 CH 1 dose a week for 1 month
You have memory loss; you are slow; you are suffering from a general slowing down (period late, educational underachievement, and so on)	Baryta carbonicum 9 CH 2 pillules 3 times a day

INDICATIONS	TREATMENT
You have been worn out for a long time with what could be called chronic slowness	Baryta carbonicum 15 CH 2 pillules 3 times a day *or* 1 dose a week
In the case of a child who is sleepy during the day, feels tired all of a sudden, lacks concentration at school, and is of the phosphoric type	Kalium phosphoricum 9 CH 2 pillules 3 times a day
In a case of physical, mental, and emotional fatigue from school work, for the carbonics; if the person is also sexually excited	Baryta carbonicum 9 CH 1 dose a week *or* Rana bufo 9 CH 1 dose a week
In the case of a student who complains of memory blocks	Kalium phosphoricum 9 CH 2 pillules 3 times a day *combined with* Phosphoricum acidum 9 CH 1 dose twice a week *or* 2 pillules 3 times a day
You have sudden bouts of tiredness, suffer from general weakness, are often cold, have brittle nails, and are of the carbonic type	Graphites 9 CH 2 pillules 3 times a day
You are a senior citizen, (especially if you have high blood pressure)	Baryta carbonicum 9 CH 2 pillules twice a day

INDICATIONS	TREATMENT
You are "knocked out" by a high fever (in the case of the flu, for example), you have difficulty opening your eyes, you tremble, but you are not thirsty	*In combination with other remedies, for muscle pain, for example* Gelsemium 5 CH 1 dose, possibly repeated the next day *or* 2 pillules 3 times a day
You become lifeless before an exam or an important event (job interview, driving test, and so on), you feel as if you were on the edge of a cliff, you cannot put your ideas together or reflect on anything, and you tremble; you feel as if your legs have been cut off, and you may have diarrhea	Gelsemium 9 CH 2 pillules the day before the exam 2 pillules 30 minutes before the exam 2 pillules (if possible) during the exam
The apathy comes on after anesthesia; you no longer feel pain; you fall asleep during the day but are wide awake in the evening	Opium 9 CH 2 pillules 3 times a day *and to "detoxify" the system, evacuate the medicinal substances* Nux vomica 5 CH 2 pillules 3 times a day
Your asthenia is due to radiation or exposure to X-rays	Radium bromatum 5 CH 2 pillules 3 times a day
You are worn out after being active; you have muscle pain	Arnica montana 9 CH 2 pillules 3 times a day *combined with* Rhus toxicodendron 9 CH 2 pillules 3 times a day

INDICATIONS	TREATMENT
You are worn out after a long journey and you have jet lag and altitude sickness	Coca 5 CH 2 pillules 3 times a day *combined with* Cocculus indicus 5 CH 2 pillules 30 minutes before leaving *and with* Melatonin 7 CH 2 pillules 30 minutes before leaving 2 pillules at the start of the journey *then* 2 pillules every 3 hours during the journey *and* 2 pillules on going to bed, once you arrive
You are overburdened with work and feel sleepy after meals, and a short siesta helps you a great deal	Nux vomica 5 CH 2 pillules 30 minutes before a meal
You feel sleepy after meals and fall asleep watching television, but anxiety prevents you from sleeping once you are in bed	Nux vomica 9 CH 2 pillules on going to bed

See also: Weakness, fatigue, burnout, page 161.

ADVICE

If you are really worn out and these remedies do not work, you should not be complacent: this symptom may be masking a deeper condition, such as depression, a serious viral infection, or even a brain tumor. Consult a doctor who could make a definite diagnosis. Homeopathy will, in any event, still be useful to make you more comfortable.

MOUTH ULCERS

Small painful ulcer on the mucous membranes in the mouth (interior of the cheeks, tongue, gums). It feels like burns in your mouth, especially on contact with acidic or salty food.

INDICATIONS	TREATMENT
The ulcer is situated on the interior of the cheeks; it is white and painful	Borax 5 CH 2 pillules 3 times a day
The mouth ulcer is slightly fissured, painful, very sensitive to heat and cold, and it bleeds	Borax 5 CH 2 pillules 3 times a day *combined with* Nitricum acidum 5 CH 2 pillules 3 times a day
The mouth ulcer is burning; it forms a large blister	Cantharis 5 CH 2 pillules 3 times a day
The ulcer is white, as is your tongue; you salivate profusely and have bad breath	Mercurius solubilis 5 CH 2 pillules 3 times a day
The mouth ulcer is fissured and bloody, and you have a white, thickened tongue	Mercurius corrosivus 5 CH 2 pillules 3 times a day *or if the pain is significant* 2 pillules 6 to 8 times a day

INDICATIONS	TREATMENT
The ulcers are more painful at night and your mouth is dark red	Lachesis 5 CH 2 pillules 3 times a day *and if you are very talkative* Lachesis 9 CH 2 pillules 3 times a day

ADVICE

Good oral hygiene can't do any harm: clean your teeth and rinse your mouth regularly. Bicarbonate mouthwashes can improve the general state of the mouth and balance its pH. You can also use Phytolacca in mother tincture or Calendula mother tincture at a rate of 10 drops in a glass of water to rinse the mouth as often as possible, or combined with Echinacea purpurea mother tincture and Hydrastis mother tincture.

APHONIA

See: Hoarseness, aphonia, page 153.

EXCESSIVE APPETITE

Excessive hunger, with constant desire to eat. You obsessively consume anything that is edible, sometimes until you feel ill.

INDICATIONS	TREATMENT
For a baby that is of the carbonic type and very greedy	Calcarea carbonicum 9 CH 1 dose a week

INDICATIONS	TREATMENT
You have an increased appetite after having stopped smoking, or you continually eat snacks to the point of getting indigestion	Antimonium crudum 9 CH 2 pillules 3 times a day
You eat snacks from boredom all day long and you are not hungry at mealtimes	Ignatia amara 5 CH 2 pillules 3 times a day
You eat to compensate for a psychological problem that you cannot express	Staphysagria 9 CH 1 dose a week
You are particularly fond of savory foods; you are thirsty and constipated; the upper part of your body remains thin while the lower part is filled out	Natrum muriaticum 9 CH 2 pillules 3 times a day
You are fond of sugary foods; you look flushed and fit and cannot cope with heat	Sulfur 5 CH 1 dose a week
You have water retention after taking cortisone for a long time	Cortisone 9 CH 1 dose a week *and to stimulate the adrenal glands* Ribes nigrum (Blackcurrant) macerate of the bud 1 DH 30 to 40 drops 3 times a day
If the water retention is generalized in your whole body	*Add to preceding treatment* Natrum sulphuricum 5 CH 2 pillules 3 times a day

INDICATIONS	TREATMENT
If the water retention affects the lower part of your body and is accompanied by cellulite	*Add, instead* Thuja occidentalis 5 CH 2 pillules 3 times a day
To diminish the appetite while on a diet	Hypophysis 9 CH 1 dose a week *alternating in the same week with* Hypothalamus 9 CH 1 dose a week
You become aggressive when you have nothing to eat; you wake up at night to eat and you eat snacks continually; you have memory loss and everything improves when you eat	Anacardium orientale 9 CH 2 pillules when you feel hungry
You are timid and apathetic, have a general slowing down of the system and, moreover, are slow to heal from wounds	Graphites 9 CH 2 pillules 3 times a day

ADVICE

Good drainage, in the form of complex remedies, generally in liquid form, is sometimes necessary before undertaking any treatment. (See: Complex remedies, drainage (Liver, kidneys, skin), page 320.)

Excessive appetite, which causes weight gain, can be the cause of many pathologies: rheumatism, cardiac problems, renal problems, hypertension. An appointment with a dietitian could get things back on track and reestablish the few basic rules for a healthy, balanced diet with the rule: "A little bit of everything, not too much in excess." Excessive appetite can also mask a psychological disorder in a person who is insecure, uses food to compensate for their insecurity, and is trying to hide behind their corpulence. Psychological help may be useful to deal with this symptom in the long term.

APPETITE (LACK OF)

Disappearance of hunger, sometimes with a feeling of disgust for food.

INDICATIONS	TREATMENT
The appetite disappears after an infectious disease (for example, a sore throat); you have had diarrhea and vomiting and feel severe fatigue	China rubra 5 CH (*Cinchona officinalis*) 2 pillules 3 times a day
You lose weight, particularly in the upper body; you only eat savory things; you are very thirsty and constipated; your lips are dry	Natrum muriaticum 5 CH 2 pillules 3 times a day, for 1 or 2 months
You feel cold and sweaty, suffer from demineralization, and are susceptible to infections	Silicea 9 CH 1 dose twice a week

INDICATIONS	TREATMENT
The appetite disappears after a vaccination or taking antibiotics	Thuja occidentalis 9 CH 1 dose the day before the vaccination 1 dose the day after the vaccination

ADVICE

If the origin of the loss of appetite is psychological, consult your doctor. They will prescribe the remedy specific to your situation. If the cause is not psychological, a healthy lifestyle could help prime the system again: walks in the open air, a little exercise, sleeping well at regular times, and a little effort in presentation of food to arouse the taste buds and the appetite. But weight loss connected to loss of appetite could be a sign of a severe illness; if it continues, it is essential to get medical advice.

OSTEOARTHRITIS

Chronic condition of joint cartilage due to aging, which could entail swelling and pain (mainly in the hips, knees, and fingers).

INDICATIONS	TREATMENT
Osteoarthritis accompanied by demineralization	Calcarea carbonica in Schuessler Tissue Salts 8 DH *and* Calcarea phosphorica in Schuessler Tissue Salts 6 DH 2 to 3 tablets 3 times a day *combined with* Silicea 6 DH 2 to 3 tablets 3 times a day

INDICATIONS	TREATMENT
You are demineralized, have dental problems (cavities), and have a tendency to stoop	*Add to the preceding remedies* Calcarea fluorica in Schuessler Tissue Salts 6 DH 2 to 3 tablets 3 times a day
You are subject to fractures	*Add* Symphytum 5 CH 2 pillules 3 times a day *combined with* Arnica montana 9 CH 2 pillules 3 times a day
You have weight problems, do not pass much urine, and are demineralized	Horsetail (*Equisetum arvense*) mother tincture 50 drops 3 times a day
Your joints are painful, you feel better when they are compressed (by a knee pad or elastic bandage, for example), and you feel better when resting	Bryonia 5 CH 2 pillules 3 times a day
The pain is less intense when you move but aggravated by damp cold	Rhus toxicodendron 5 CH 2 pillules 3 times a day
The pain is very severe	Ribes nigrum mother tincture 20 drops 3 times a day *combined with* Harpagophytum (Devil's Claw) mother tincture 20 drops 3 times a day

INDICATIONS	TREATMENT
The osteoarthritis is accompanied by stiffness	Tuberculinum residuum 5 CH 2 pillules 3 times a day *combined with* Causticum 5 CH 2 pillules 3 times a day
The osteoarthritis is accompanied by small bony excrescences	Hekla lava 5 CH 2 pillules 3 times a day *combined with* Calcarea fluorica 9 CH 2 pillules 3 times a day
The osteoarthritis is accompanied by an accumulation of uric acid in the joints	Uricum acidum 5 CH 2 pillules 3 times a day *combined with* Erigeron canadensis mother tincture 20 drops 3 times a day
The osteoarthritis is accompanied by infectious rheumatism and burning diarrhea	Sulphur iodatum 5 CH 2 pillules 3 times a day

ADVICE

Being overweight can aggravate pathologies associated with osteoarthritis. The first recommendation is to try to lose a little weight. (See: Excessive appetite, page 78.) Do not force the joints affected by osteoarthritis: that will only aggravate the inflammation. Avoid stairs and high heels, violent sports, and walking long distances if the knee is affected.

ASTHENIA

See: Apathy, asthenia, dejection, page 73.

ASTHMA

Respiratory problems and difficulty exhaling, mainly due to bronchial spasms caused by allergy with edema, vexation or stress, or a bacterial or microscopic fungal infection, manifest as asthma attacks. In certain forms of serious asthma, you find a combination of bronchial constriction, edema, and infection.

INDICATIONS	TREATMENT
TO TREAT THE ATTACK	
If the bronchi are very much affected, if the attack is triggered by an allergy	Lung histamine 5 CH 2 pillules 3 to 4 times a day *(or more, if necessary)*
To minimize the attack	Ethyl sulfur dichloratum 5 CH 2 pillules 3 times a day *(or more, if necessary)*
In the case of allergy causing edema in the bronchi	Apis mellifica 5 CH 2 pillules 3 times a day *(or more, if necessary)*
The attack is due to an allergy to house dust or dust mites	Blatta orientalis 5 CH 2 pillules 3 times a day
The attack is aggravated by humidity	Aralia racemosa 5 CH 2 pillules 3 times a day
During the attack the face of the person affected becomes blue and they cannot breathe	*Perhaps while awaiting the arrival of the ambulance* Cuprum metallicum 5 CH 2 pillules every 10 minutes
The attack is accompanied by bouts of nocturnal coughs	Drosera 5 CH 2 pillules 3 times a day

INDICATIONS	TREATMENT
The attack is in a child, whose nose is blocked and who snores, night and day	Sambucus nigra 5 CH 2 pillules 3 times a day *combined with* Cuprum metallicum 5 CH 2 pillules 3 times a day
The child is puny and subject to ear, nose, and throat infections	*Combine with* Aviaire 5 CH 2 pillules 3 times a day
The attack, ameliorated by fresh air, affects an elderly person who feels too weak even to fan themselves and asks someone to do it for them	Carbo vegetabilis 5 CH 2 pillules 3 times a day
FOR DEEP-ACTING TREATMENT	
Your attacks come on between 1 and 3 a.m.; you are asthenic but agitated, anxious, and sickly; ameliorated by fresh air	Arsenicum album 9 CH *or if there are mental/emotional problems* Arsenicum album 15 CH 2 pillules on going to bed 2 pillules at the time of the attack
Your attacks come on between 2 and 4 a.m.; you are worn out to the point of staying sitting on your bed, unable to get up	Kalium carbonicum 9 CH *or if there are mental/emotional problems* 2 pillules on going to bed 2 pillules at the time of the attack
The attack comes on at mealtimes	Antimonium crudum 9 CH 2 pillules 3 times a day
The attack comes on just after a meal	Nux vomica 7 CH 2 pillules 3 times a day

INDICATIONS	TREATMENT
You are agitated; you crave sugar although it aggravates your asthma	Argentum nitricum 9 CH 2 pillules 3 times a day
Your asthma is aggravated by humidity	Dulcamara 5 CH 2 pillules 3 times a day *combined with* Natrum sulphuricum 5 CH 2 pillules 3 times a day
You feel better out at sea and worse as soon as you arrive back on land	Bromum 7 CH 2 pillules 3 times a day *or* Medorrhinum 7 CH 2 pillules 3 times a day
You feel worse by the sea	Natrum muriaticum 9 CH 2 pillules 3 times a day
You suffer repeatedly from bronchitis, you have difficulty in expectorating but feel better after coughing, and your tongue is thick and white	Antimonium tartaricum 5 CH 2 pillules 3 times a day
You smoke and cough	Tabacum 5 CH 2 pillules 3 times a day *combined with* Lobelia inflata 5 CH 2 pillules 3 times a day
The attack causes a cough and nausea; your tongue is "clean"	Ipecac 5 CH 2 pillules 3 times a day

INDICATIONS	TREATMENT
The asthma is caused by a malfunction of the adrenal glands (after treatment with cortisone, for example), and you suffer from water retention	Natrum sulphuricum 5 CH 2 pillules 3 times a day *combined with* Cortisone 9 CH 2 pillules 3 times a day *and with* liver and kidney drainage *(See: Complex remedies, page 320)* 20 drops 3 times a day
The asthma appears after a vaccination or antibiotherapy	Thuja occidentalis 5 CH 2 pillules 3 times a day
The asthma appears after BCG vaccination	Thuja occidentalis 5 CH 2 pillules 3 times a day *combined with* VAB 9 CH 2 pillules 3 times a day

ADVICE

If the asthma is of allergenic origin, you need to do everything possible to avoid all the substances that cause the allergies. If you know what your particular enemy is, the task will be easier. If this is not the case, an allergist could identify it and make it easier to prevent the allergy. You could have isotherapy prescribed for the allergen responsible for your attack (See: Allergies, page 61).

POSTPARTUM DEPRESSION

See: Pregnancy, page 181.

BLOATING

See: Flatulence (eructations, burps), bloating, page 56.

BRUISE, HEMATOMA

Painful, superficial reaction after a blow or a trauma, accompanied by a change of skin color (which could turn blue or reddish-violet). The bruise appears very quickly after the blow, due to the rupture of small blood vessels that release an effusion of blood under the skin, and it is very sensitive to the touch.

INDICATIONS	TREATMENT
For bruising on the body	*If the trauma is very localized* Arnica montana 5 CH 2 pillules just after the trauma *or if the trauma causes a number of hematomas* Arnica montana 9 CH 2 pillules just after the trauma
In the case of a black eye or one that is covered in bruising where the pain improves with the application of ice	Arnica montana 5 CH 2 pillules just after the trauma *combined with* Ledum palustre 5 CH 2 pillules just after the trauma
Bruising appears spontaneously, without any trauma	Lachesis 9 CH 2 pillules 3 times a day

INDICATIONS	TREATMENT
For mental/emotional trauma (in the case of mental/emotional shock or the emotional state resulting from a trauma)	Arnica montana 15 CH 2 pillules after the trauma

ADVICE

The spontaneous appearance of bruising may be the symptom of a liver problem or alcoholism. Medical advice will potentially prove necessary. For small bruises that are not serious and are common in childhood, a big hug and tender affection with a compress soaked in Arnica montana mother tincture are recommended.

INJURY/SWELLING

Rounded, painful swelling that appears following a hit or a violent blow, especially if it is on the head and the forehead.

INDICATIONS	TREATMENT
Once the swelling has started	Arnica montana 5 CH 2 pillules just after the trauma *or* 1 dose just after the trauma

INDICATIONS	TREATMENT
The pain improves with cold or application of ice	Arnica montana 5 CH 2 pillules just after the trauma *combined with* Ledum palustre 5 CH 2 pillules just after the trauma *and possibly* Apis mellifica 5 CH 2 pillules 3 times a day
The pain improves when you apply pressure to the swelling with the hand or with a coin	Arnica montana 5 CH 2 pillules just after the trauma *combined with* Bryonia 5 CH 2 pillules 3 times a day
The swelling has formed	Arnica montana 5 CH 2 pillules just after the trauma *combined with* Hekla lava 5 CH 2 pillules 3 times a day
You keep injuring yourself	Arnica montana 5 CH 2 pillules just after the trauma *combined with* Calcarea fluorica 9 CH 2 pillules 3 times a day

ADVICE

To avoid the injury swelling too much, you should take Arnica montana 5 CH as soon as possible after the trauma and apply ice or compress the swelling with a handkerchief or a scarf, leaning heavily on it.

BUZZING AND RINGING IN THE EAR (TINNITUS)

Continuous, dull sounds heard in the ears, mainly when it is silent or very calm.

INDICATIONS	TREATMENT
The buzzing is incessant and accompanied by diminished hearing capacity	China rubra 5 CH (*Cinchona officinalis*) 2 pillules 3 times a day
The buzzing is triggered by serous otitis (inflammation of the middle ear)	*To protect the Eustachian tube* Mercurius dulcis 5 CH 2 pillules 3 times a day *alternating with* Kalium muriaticum 5 CH 2 pillules 3 times a day
The buzzing comes on after taking quinine, aspirin, or antibiotics and noticeably diminishes hearing capacity	Chininum salicylicum 5 CH 2 pillules 3 times a day *or* Chininum arsenicosum 5 CH 2 pillules 3 times a day *combined with* Thuja occidentalis 5 CH 2 pillules 3 times a day *and* Streptomycinum 5 CH 2 pillules 3 times a day
The buzzing is triggered by a medicine	Isotherapic of the medicine 5 CH 2 pillules 3 times a day

An ear, nose, and throat examination is essential in all cases: buzzing in the ears can be a symptom of hypertension, a vascular problem, or a disorder of the nervous system. Homeopathy can be used only if all possibility of serious illness has been ruled out, or in addition to conventional treatment.

COLD SORES

See: Herpes, page 189.

BRONCHITIS

Inflammation of the bronchi due to virus or bacteria. You cough and have difficulty breathing, you have a burning sensation in your chest, and you are feverish.

INDICATIONS	TREATMENT
You have difficulty coughing, but expectoration helps	Antimonium tartaricum 5 CH 2 pillules 3 times a day *combined with* Pyrogenium 9 CH 2 pillules 3 times a day
You are nauseated, your tongue remains clean, and you do not feel better after vomiting	Ipecac 5 CH 2 pillules 3 times a day
The bronchitis causes asthma-like spasms	Cuprum metallicum 5 CH 2 pillules 3 times a day

INDICATIONS	TREATMENT
The bronchitis causes bouts of coughing at night	Drosera 5 CH 2 pillules 3 times a day
You have a dry cough, difficulty breathing, a fever, and slight anemia	Ferrum phosphoricum 5 CH 2 pillules 3 times a day
The bronchitis is aggravated by house dust, dust mites, or damp cold; it causes a kind of asthma attack	Blatta orientalis 5 CH 2 pillules 3 times a day
You have difficulty coughing	Ethyl sulfur dichloratum 5 CH 2 pillules 3 times a day
There is considerable edema in the bronchi, and you are tired	Kalium carbonicum 5 CH 2 pillules 3 times a day
There is considerable edema in the bronchi; you are tired, and you have great difficulty breathing	Ammonium carbonicum 5 CH 2 pillules 3 times a day
For children with respiratory weakness	*Combine with* Aviaire 5 CH 2 pillules 3 times a day
The bronchitis is accompanied by yellowish, non-irritating secretions, aggravated by cold but better in fresh air	Pulsatilla 5 CH 2 pillules 3 times a day

INDICATIONS	TREATMENT
You smoke	*While waiting to give up the habit* Tabacum 5 CH 2 pillules 3 times a day *combined with* Lobelia inflata 5 CH 2 pillules 3 times a day
IN ALL CASES	
A good drainage remedy may improve the symptoms	Natrum sulphuricum 5 CH 2 pillules 3 times a day *combined with* Quebracho 5 CH 2 pillules 3 times a day *or* Orthosiphon mother tincture 20 drops 3 times a day
If there is edema	Apis mellifica 5 CH 2 pillules 3 times a day
To drain the respiratory tract	Yerba santa 5 CH 2 pillules 3 times a day *combined with* Quebracho 3 CH 2 pillules 3 times a day

ADVICE

Do you smoke? It is time to stop!

Antibiotics are sometimes essential (but not always) to treat bronchitis, especially in the elderly, who risk significant complications.

BRONCHIOLITIS

The asthma-like type of bronchitis in young children causes a very intense cough and considerable respiratory problems. Bronchiolitis affects mainly children under age 2, often when there are epidemics in the winter.

INDICATIONS	TREATMENT
The child has difficulty coughing	Ethyl sulfur dichloratum 5 CH 2 pillules 3 times a day
The child has spasms	Cuprum metallicum 5 CH 2 pillules 3 times a day
The child has nausea	Ipecac 5 CH 2 pillules 3 times a day
The bronchiolitis is aggravated by pollution	Peak Time Pollution 3 5 CH 2 pillules 3 times a day
The child is agitated and anxious	Arsenicum album 9 CH 2 pillules at the time of the respiratory problems
What is more, the child suffers from respiratory weakness	*Combine with the preceding remedy* Aviaire 5 CH 2 pillules 3 times a day
If there is edema of the respiratory tract	Apis mellifica 5 CH 2 pillules 3 times a day *or* Natrum sulphuricum 5 CH 2 pillules 3 times a day
To stimulate the adrenal glands	Ribes nigrum, tincture of macerated bud 1 DH 20 drops morning and midday

Respiratory physiotherapy is a necessary treatment for bronchiolitis: it brings great benefits in helping the child to breathe. Avoid smoking near the child.

BURNS

Lesions of the skin and tissues of the epidermis caused by a source of heat, a flame, or an electric current. The epidermis is red, very painful, and sensitive to touch. Depending on the degree of the burn, the skin may become purplish, with more or less extensive blistering.

INDICATIONS	TREATMENT
The skin is dry, painful, red, and hot	Belladonna 5 CH 2 pillules 3 times a day *combined with* Calendula cream *or* Local application of Bellis perennis mother tincture
The burn causes edema, and the pain is better with cold (application of ice, for example)	Apis mellifica 5 CH 2 pillules 3 times a day
The burn causes small blisters that are very irritating	Urtica urens 5 CH 2 pillules 3 times a day
The burn causes large blisters	Cantharis 5 CH 2 pillules 3 times a day

INDICATIONS	TREATMENT
IN ALL CASES	
Local application of	Calendula mother tincture
	Bellis perennis oil
	Centella asiatica 5% cream
	Mimosa tenuiflora 5% cream
	or
	a combination of these active principles

ADVICE

As soon as you have a burn, hold the whole area affected under really cold water for some time. This cooling will diminish the painful sensation by anesthetizing the area concerned and prevent the burn from extending too far. But do not place ice cubes or butter directly on the lesion: this would only make it worse.

In the case of extensive or substantial burns, go to the hospital to avoid the risk of infection.

CALCULI

Hard formations (that look like stones) that impede a channel (such as the urethra or a urinary duct) or that are in an organ (such as kidney, gall bladder, salivary glands) and may entail pain and colic (hepatic or renal). It is always helpful to understand the nature of a calculus to determine how to address the problem.

INDICATIONS	TREATMENT
The calculus causes painful spasms; you feel better when you bend over	Magnesia phosphorica 5 CH 2 pillules 3 times a day *combined with* Colocynth 5 CH 2 pillules 3 times a day
The calculus causes painful spasms; you feel better when you stretch out	Dioscorea villosa 5 CH 2 pillules 3 times a day
The calculus is due to excess uric acid	Uricum acidum 5 CH 2 pillules 3 times a day
The calculus is due to excess oxalic acid or calcium	Oxalalicum acidum 5 CH 2 pillules 3 times a day *combined with* Calcarea carbonica 5 CH 2 pillules 3 times a day
The calculus causes irritation and burns before, during, and after each micturition, sometimes with bleeding	*While waiting to consult a doctor* Cantharis 5 CH 2 pillules 3 times a day
The calculus causes inflammation and problems urinating	Apis mellifica 9 CH 2 pillules 3 times a day

INDICATIONS	TREATMENT
The calculus causes an infection	Colibacillinum 9 CH (*Bacillus coli*)
	2 pillules 3 times a day
	and
	Serum Anticolibacillosis 8 DH
	1 vial a day
	combined with Formica rufa composite
	5 to 10 drops 3 times a day
	and with
	Cantharis 5 CH
	2 pillules 3 times a day

ADVICE

It is useful to know the nature of the calculus and its significance when choosing a treatment. Calculi sometimes need surgical intervention, although these days many can be treated with ultrasound. Seek medical advice.

CAVITIES

Cavities that form in a tooth following the destruction of the enamel and the dentin. A cavity can be very painful.

INDICATIONS	TREATMENT
In case of cavities	Calcarea fluorica 9 CH
	2 pillules 3 times a day
	or
	1 dose twice a week
	combined with
	Silicea 5 CH
	2 pillules 3 times a day

INDICATIONS	TREATMENT
If the tooth with a cavity smells bad	Kreosotum 5 CH 2 pillules 3 times a day
To prevent cavities	*To better assimilate fluoride from food* Calcarea fluorica 9 CH 1 dose a week
Black cavities situated at the neck of the teeth (where the tooth meets the gum)	Kreosotum 5 CH

ADVICE

It is essential to see a dentist! Brush teeth thoroughly and avoid consumption of candy, sweet foods, and soda. Note that taking an excessive quantity of fluoride tablets can have side effects (poisoning or making the teeth fragile).

CATARACTS

Opacity of the lens of the eye leading to partial or even total blindness.

INDICATIONS	TREATMENT
In all cases	Naphtalinum 5 CH 2 pillules 3 times a day *combined with* Thiosinaminum 5 CH 2 pillules 3 times a day *and* Causticum 5 CH 2 pillules 3 times a day

Surgery is always necessary. It is very effective, and these days, it is becoming less and less traumatic.

CELLULITE

Fat that has accumulated under the skin. Your thighs and buttocks look like an orange peel and are painful with pressure.

INDICATIONS	TREATMENT
For standard cellulite in the areas of the thighs and buttocks	Thuja occidentalis 5 CH 2 pillules 3 times a day
For cellulite all over the body	Natrum sulphuricum 5 CH 2 pillules 3 times a day
For painful and inflamed cellulite	Cantharis 5 CH 2 pillules 3 times a day
For drainage	Orthosiphon mother tincture 20 drops 3 times a day or Berberis vulgaris 5 CH 2 pillules 3 times a day

ADVICE

To help counteract cellulite, have a healthy diet, don't eat too much fat, drink plenty of fluids, and be active.

GREASY HAIR

Tendency for hair to become greasy and heavy. It doesn't matter how much you wash it, your hair always looks wet and sticky.

INDICATIONS	TREATMENT
Your hair is very greasy	Sulfur 5 CH 2 pillules 3 times a day *combined with* Uriage Thermal Spring Water 5 CH 2 pillules 3 times a day
Your hair is very greasy and tends to fall out; you have dandruff and feel tired	Selenium 5 CH 2 pillules 3 times a day
You have dandruff and eczema that make the scalp itch	Arsenicum album 5 CH 2 pillules 3 times a day
You also have acne	Kalium bromatum 5 CH 2 pillules 3 times a day *combined with* Staphylococcinum 9 CH 2 pillules 3 times a day *and with* Hepar sulphur 4 CH 2 pillules 3 times a day
You are an adolescent, and your hair becomes even greasier before your period	Folliculinum 9 CH 1 dose on the 14th day of the cycle *and* 1 dose on the 21st day of the cycle

See also: Hair falling out, page 106.

Do not use shampoo that is too harsh, even those recommended for greasy hair: they only have a temporary effect and by mistreating the scalp cause additional secretions, which "grease" the hair again even more quickly. Aerate your hair and brush it regularly in all directions.

DULL, BRITTLE HAIR

Tendency of hair to be dry and brittle, a little coarse to touch.

INDICATIONS	TREATMENT
You are timid	Graphites 5 CH 2 pillules 3 times a day
Your hair alternates between dry and greasy	Thuja occidentalis 5 CH 2 pillules 3 times a day
Your skin is also dry	Alumina 5 CH 2 pillules 3 times a day
Your hair is fragile and falling out	Selenium 5 CH 2 pillules 3 times a day *combined with* Thallium aceticum 5 CH 2 pillules 3 times a day

See also: Hair falling out, page 106.

ADVICE

Avoid shampoos that dry the hair and hairspray and gels that prevent the hair from breathing. Drink a lot of liquids.

EMOTIONAL SHOCK

Mental/emotional trauma, which may be caused by psychological conditions: depression after bereavement, anxiety after an accident, insomnia after good or bad news, overexcitement after passing an exam.

INDICATIONS	TREATMENT
You tremble	Gelsemium 9 CH 2 pillules 3 times a day
You have lost someone close to you	Ignatia amara 9 CH 2 pillules 3 times a day
You are agitated and impatient	Argentum nitricum 9 CH 2 pillules 3 times a day
You are hyperactive	Nux vomica 9 CH 2 pillules 3 times a day
Shock after a happy event and loss of sleep	Coffea 7 CH 2 pillules in the evening
IN ALL CASES	
After any emotional or traumatic shock	Arnica montana 9 CH 2 pillules 3 times a day
Anger that is not expressed	Staphysagria 9 CH 2 pillules 3 times a day

ADVICE

To control problems arising from emotional storms, try relaxation techniques such as deep breathing exercises and yoga.

HAIR FALLING OUT

Progressive or sudden hair loss that could lead to complete baldness. Natural and progressive hair loss may be due to aging or genetic predisposition. Sudden hair loss, or alopecia, may be linked to strong emotion, an infection, or chemotherapy.

INDICATIONS	TREATMENT
For any hair loss	Thallium aceticum 5 CH 2 pillules 3 times a day *alternating with* Selenium 5 CH 2 pillules 3 times a day
You have combination skin and your hair is greasy in places	Thuja occidentalis 5 CH 2 pillules 3 times a day
Hair loss is due to medicines (e.g., chemotherapy)	Isotherapic of the medicine 5 CH 2 pillules 3 times a day
Your hair loss is due to radiation therapy or exposure to X-rays	Radium bromatum 5 CH 2 pillules 3 times a day
Your hair falls out and is prematurely white	Lycopodium 5 CH 2 pillules 3 times a day
Your hair falls out after a shock or emotion	Arnica montana 9 CH 2 pillules 3 times a day
Your hair falls out after excessive mental stimulation or because you are tired on a mental/emotional level	Phosphoricum acidum 9 CH 2 pillules 3 times a day *combined with* Kalium phosphoricum 5 CH 2 pillules 3 times a day

ADVICE

Hair falling out due to aging is a natural phenomenon, some-times genetic, and very difficult to prevent. Even if it may seem aesthetically unpleasing and be difficult to tolerate, it should not be the cause of any anxiety about your health.

On the other hand, in the event of sudden hair loss that cannot be explained, it is essential to seek medical advice. It could be masking a serious infection, a fungal condition, or some other cause that calls for diagnosis and appropriate treatment.

SCARRING

Mark left on the skin by a lesion, wound, burn, cut, spot, or surgical operation. Scarring may take different forms—red or purplish mark, white line, excrescence, bulge, mottling—and it is rarely attractive.

INDICATIONS	TREATMENT
The scarring is due to a burn	Cantharis 5 CH 2 pillules 3 times a day
The scarring is due to a cut (knife, scissors, or lancet after an operation)	Staphysagria 5 CH 2 pillules 3 times a day
The scarring is due to a puncture wound (vaccination, acupuncture, or insect sting)	Hypericum perforatum 5 CH 2 pillules 3 times a day
The scarring is red	Belladonna 5 CH 2 pillules 3 times a day

INDICATIONS	TREATMENT
The scarring forms a kind of raised shape (keloid scarring)	Graphites 5 CH 2 pillules 3 times a day *combined with* Silicea 5 CH 2 pillules 3 times a day
The scarring is keloid and burning	Radium bromatum 5 CH 2 pillules 3 times a day
To restore elasticity to the skin in the scarred area	Calendula ointment local application *combined with* Local application of Centella asiatica mother tincture *and* Local application of Mimosa tenuiflora mother tincture

ADVICE

After a cut or any other incision of the skin, you need to immediately disinfect and thoroughly clean the wound to avoid leaving the smallest foreign body in it and prevent the formation of scars.

CIRCULATION (PROBLEMS WITH), VARICOSE VEINS, HEAVY LEGS, HEMORRHOIDS

Increase in volume or slowing of the blood flow. Circulation problems cause a variety of disturbances. You may suffer from swollen, heavy legs, pain in veins and phlebitis, varicose dilations, hemorrhoids.

INDICATIONS	TREATMENT
You suffer from prolapse of the organs associated with your bad circulation, and brisk exercise does you good	Sepia 9 CH 2 pillules in the evening on going to bed 2 pillules at about 11 a.m.
To liquefy the blood and diminish coagulation time	Bothrops 5 CH 2 pillules 3 times a day
To promote circulation	Hamamelis 4 DH 10 drops 3 times a day *or* a complex remedy with Hamamelis, Corylus avellana, Ginkgo biloba, Red vine *(See: Complex remedies, page 320)* 10 drops 3 times a day
You develop spontaneous hematomas and cannot wear either stockings or belts	Lachesis 9 CH 2 pillules 3 times a day *combined with* Arnica montana 9 CH 2 pillules 3 times a day
You are an adolescent, you have bad circulation, your ankles are mottled, and you feel better when walking in the fresh air	Pulsatilla 9 CH 2 pillules 3 times a day

INDICATIONS	TREATMENT
VARICOSE VEINS	
In all cases	Arnica montana 9 CH 2 pillules 3 times a day *combined with* Vipera redi 5 CH 2 pillules 3 times a day Hamamelis 5 CH 2 pillules 3 times a day
You have a tendency to varicose ulcers	Fluoricum acidum 9 CH 2 pillules 3 times a day
You have venous congestion in your legs	Aesculus hippocastanum 5 CH 2 pillules 3 times a day
HEAVY LEGS	
You have heavy legs with restlessness in the limbs	Zincum metallicum 9 CH 2 pillules 3 times a day
You have heavy legs, and you feel better with the legs raised	Vipera redi 9 CH 2 pillules 3 times a day
You are pregnant; you have hemorrhoids and heavy legs	Collinsonia canadensis 9 CH 2 pillules 3 times a day
In case of venous insufficiency	*Add to preceding remedies* Calcarea fluorica 9 CH 1 dose a week

INDICATIONS	TREATMENT
HEMORRHOIDS	
The hemorrhoids are large and red	Aesculus hippocastanum 5 CH 2 pillules 3 times a day *combined with* Hamamelis 5 CH 2 pillules 3 times a day *and with* Ginkgo biloba mother tincture *In case of acute onset* 50 drops 3 times a day *Maintenance* 10 to 15 drops 3 times a day
The hemorrhoids bleed	Mercurius corrosivus 5 CH 2 pillules 3 times a day *or* Fluoricum acidum 5 CH 2 pillules 3 times a day
The hemorrhoids are ulcerated	Muriaticum acidum 5 CH 2 pillules 3 times a day
The hemorrhoids weep slightly and you have the sensation of a splinter pain before and after defecating	Paeonia 5 CH 2 pillules 3 times a day
The hemorrhoids cause serious burning pain	Capsicum 5 CH 2 pillules 3 times a day
You have involuntary stools	Aloe 5 CH 2 pillules 3 times a day
You eat too much, abuse alcohol, and are sedentary	Nux vomica 5 CH 2 pillules 3 times a day

INDICATIONS	TREATMENT
You are an alcoholic, your blood does not coagulate, you tremble, and you are generally in a bad state	Sulphuricum acidum 5 CH 2 pillules 3 times a day

ADVICE

Avoid staying in a standing or sitting position for a long time, taking baths that are too hot and dilate the veins, or wearing tight clothing. Do some exercise, like going for a walk or a swim.

COLIC

Violent abdominal pain. You suffer from cramp-like spasms and often diarrhea.

Colic can be renal (when it is associated with the presence of calculi in the urinary ducts) or hepatic (where the biliary ducts are involved). Mental/emotional events are sometimes the cause of an attack.

INDICATIONS	TREATMENT
To soothe the spasms, especially if they are less painful when you bend over	Magnesia phosphorica 5 CH 2 pillules 3 times a day
To help the pain caused by the spasms	Cuprum metallicum 5 CH 2 pillules 3 times a day
The colic is caused by apprehension about an alarming event or by indignation	Colocynthis 9 CH 2 pillules 3 times a day

INDICATIONS	TREATMENT
The colic is due to food poisoning and you feel better with a hot water bottle	Arsenicum album 5 CH 2 pillules 3 times a day
The colic is due to eating fruits that are acidic/not ripe enough	Rheum 5 CH 2 pillules 3 times a day
The colic causes gushing, liquid diarrhea	Podophyllum peltatum 9 CH 2 pillules 3 times a day
The colic causes exhausting diarrhea	China rubra 5 CH (*Cinchona officinalis*) 2 pillules 3 times a day
The colic causes diarrhea accompanied by perspiration and malaise, which can even lead to fainting	Veratrum album 5 CH 2 pillules 3 times a day
The colic causes diarrhea with flatulence and ketoacidosis	Senna 5 CH 2 pillules 3 times a day
The colic causes diarrhea that can make you bad-tempered	Chamomilla 9 CH 2 pillules 3 times a day

See also: Calculi, page 98; Diarrhea, page 135.

ADVICE

During an attack of colic:

- Avoid any travel by car and try to rest.

- Avoid putting cold applications, such as bags of ice, on the abdomen; have a hot bath instead.

- Avoid drinking.

CONJUNCTIVITIS

Inflammation characterized by redness of the conjunctiva, the membrane surrounding the eye. Your eyes are bloodshot, you are sensitive to light, and your eye is sometimes swollen and irritated and watery.

INDICATIONS	TREATMENT
Your eye is irritated and inflamed with profuse tearing	Euphrasia 5 CH 2 pillules 3 times a day
Your eye is red and burning, you are sensitive to bright lights, and your pupils are dilated	Belladonna 5 CH 2 pillules 3 times a day
There is a yellowish discharge from the eye	Hydrastis 5 CH 2 pillules 3 times a day
The discharge is non-irritating	Pulsatilla 5 CH 2 pillules 3 times a day
The discharge is viscous and forms crusts	Kalium bichromicum 5 CH 2 pillules 3 times a day
The discharge is greenish	Mercurius solubilis 5 CH 2 pillules 3 times a day
There is slight edema at the internal corner of the eye	Kalium carbonicum 5 CH 2 pillules 3 times a day
There is slight edema in the eyelid	Apis mellifica 9 CH 2 pillules 3 times a day
Ulcerations form at the margin of the eye	Mercurius corrosivus 5 CH 2 pillules 3 times a day

INDICATIONS	TREATMENT
The conjunctivitis is the result of an allergy	Histaminum 5 CH 2 pillules 3 times a day *combined with* Isotherapic of the allergen 5 CH 2 pillules 3 times a day

ADVICE

Conjunctivitis is not a harmless condition. It is viral and very contagious, can cause keratitis or ulcerations of the cornea, and can prove very dangerous for the eye. Homeopathy should only be used in the case of benign conjunctivitis. It would be prudent to always ask an ophthalmologist for a diagnosis.

CONSTIPATION

Difficulty or impossibility passing stool. Stools are hard, dry, and passed in small quantity.

INDICATIONS	TREATMENT
You have dry skin and dry, fissured lips; you desire savory foods and have very hard stools and a tendency to demineralization.	Natrum muriaticum 5 CH 2 pillules 3 times a day
You have dry, very delicate skin; your digestive mucous membranes are dry, as is your mouth, particularly if you are elderly	Alumina 5 CH 2 pillules 3 times a day

INDICATIONS	TREATMENT
You are chilly, with dryness and fissures in the anus and a burning sensation	Graphites 5 CH 2 pillules 3 times a day
You are very thirsty and you are somewhat constipated	Bryonia 5 CH 2 pillules 3 times a day
Your constipation is intractable and accompanied by weakness of the anal muscles	Opium 5 CH 2 pillules 3 times a day
You have pains and spasms as with colic, but you cannot pass a stool	Plumbum 5 CH 2 pillules 3 times a day
You have tenesmus (empty urging to stool)	Nux vomica 5 CH 2 pillules 3 times a day
You have hemorrhoids that bleed easily	Collinsonia canadensis 5 CH 2 pillules 3 times a day
For women who get constipated when they travel	Platina 5 CH 2 pillules 3 times a day

ADVICE

A good, healthy diet can resolve many cases of constipation. This means eating fiber, green vegetables, fruit, whole-grain cereals with bran, limited quantities of white rice and bananas, and drinking a lot of fluids. Go for walks and develop your abdominal muscles.

Avoid laxatives, which irritate the intestines.

CORYZA, RHINITIS, COLDS

Infectious or allergic nasal discharge. Your nose runs and feels irritated; you sneeze and blow your nose a lot. It is a common and benign ailment of autumn and winter.

INDICATIONS	TREATMENT
The coryza is due to exposure to dry cold	Aconitum napellus 5 CH 2 pillules 3 times a day
It is due to exposure to humidity	Dulcamara 5 CH 2 pillules 3 times a day
It is due to an allergy	Histaminum 5 CH 2 pillules 3 times a day *or* Isotherapic of the allergen 5 CH 2 pillules 3 times a day
The attack is due to an allergy to house dust and/or to dust mites	Blatta orientalis 5 CH 2 pillules 3 times a day
It is due to an allergy to pollen, grass, trees, and the like.	Pollen 5 CH 2 pillules 3 times a day
The discharge resembles water, and you pick your nose	Allium cepa 5 CH 2 pillules 3 times a day
The discharge resembles water, and your eyes are irritated	Euphrasia 5 CH 2 pillules 3 times a day
The discharge resembles water, and your eyes and nose are irritated	Naphtalinum 5 CH 2 pillules 3 times a day

INDICATIONS	TREATMENT
The discharge resembles water, it is irritating, and you sneeze	Aralia racemosa 5 CH 2 pillules 3 times a day
The discharge resembles water and is accompanied by asthmatic cough; coughing spasm	Badiaga 5 CH 2 pillules 3 times a day
The discharge is yellow and irritating	Hydrastis 5 CH 2 pillules 3 times a day
The discharge is yellow and non-irritating	Pulsatilla 5 CH 2 pillules 3 times a day
The discharge is greenish	Mercurius solubilis 5 CH 2 pillules 3 times a day
The discharge is viscous and forms crusts, sometimes bloody ones	Kalium bichromicum 5 CH 2 pillules 3 times a day
The nose runs in the day and is blocked at night	Nux vomica 5 CH 2 pillules 3 times a day
The nose is blocked, particularly at night, and you have difficulty breathing	Ammonium carbonicum 5 CH 2 pillules 3 times a day
The nose is constantly blocked	Sambucus nigra 5 CH 2 pillules 3 times a day
The nose is blocked, in spite of your sneezing; you have a dry, wheezy cough	Ammonium carbonicum 5 CH 2 pillules 3 times a day

INDICATIONS	TREATMENT
Your cold causes fits of sneezing	Sabadilla 5 CH 2 pillules 3 times a day
Your cold causes a dry cough, difficulty breathing, and slight anemia	Ferrum phosphoricum 5 CH 2 pillules 3 times a day
Your cold is better by the sea or in damp weather	Medorrhinum 5 CH 2 pillules 3 times a day
You have swollen glands; you are agitated and often too hot	Sulphur iodatum 5 CH 2 pillules 3 times a day
IN CASE OF ALLERGIC RHINITIS	
In all cases	*Add* Histaminum 5 CH 2 pillules 3 times a day
You have difficulty breathing	*Add, instead* Lung histamine 5 CH 2 pillules 3 times a day
To stimulate the immune defense	Thymuline 5 CH 2 pillules 3 times a day

See also: Allergies, page 61; Sneezing, page 158.

ADVICE

It is neither unusual nor anything to worry about if you catch two or three colds every year. And when it's your turn, avoid drafts, but air out your house every day and blow your nose gently to avoid bursting the blood vessels in the nose and causing nosebleeds. You should not necessarily stay confined in a warm house, but avoid too great extremes of temperature.

BLOW, SHOCK, TRAUMA

Sudden, violent attack on one part of your body. You bump into something, you fall, you are directly hit by something that was thrown at you, and you experience bruising, hematomas, swelling, pain, and sometimes bleeding.

INDICATIONS	TREATMENT
In all cases	Arnica montana 9 CH 1 dose just after the shock
THEN ACCORDING TO THE CASE	
The blow is to the back	*Add* Dioscorea villosa 5 CH 2 pillules 3 times a day
The shock affects the eye	*To avoid a black eye, add* Ledum palustre 5 CH 2 pillules 3 times a day
The blow is to the breast	*Add* Bellis perennis 5 CH 2 pillules 3 times a day
The blow is to the tendon	*Add* Ruta graveolens 5 CH 2 pillules 3 times a day
The injury is to the neck	*For the vertebrae, add* Actaea racemosa 5 CH 2 pillules 3 times a day *and for the trapezius muscles (neck muscles), add* Lachnanthes tinctoria 5 CH 2 pillules 3 times a day

INDICATIONS	TREATMENT
The injury is from a sharp object	*Add* Hypericum perforatum 5 CH 2 pillules 3 times a day
The injury is due to a cutting object	*Add* Staphysagria 5 CH 2 pillules 3 times a day

See also: Bruise, hematoma, page 89; Injury/swelling, page 90.

ADVICE

A blow or traumatic injury may have long-term effects or consequences that are not immediately obvious. If the pain is very severe or persists, do not risk ignoring the possibility of a fracture or injury to an internal organ: seek medical advice!

SUNBURN

Burn due to too much exposure to the sun. Your skin becomes red and hot, constricted, and burning; then, after some time, it dries, goes dead, and peels, leaving a rose-colored mark and completely new skin that is more fragile and sensitive to the sun.

INDICATIONS	TREATMENT
Your skin is red, hot, and painful; you have dry mucous membranes; you are thirsty; and your pupils are dilated	Belladonna 5 CH 2 pillules 3 times a day

INDICATIONS	TREATMENT
The sunburn causes hot, painful edema soothed by cool applications; you are not thirsty and don't urinate much	Apis mellifica 9 CH 2 pillules 3 times a day
The burn causes large blisters	Cantharis 5 CH 2 pillules 3 times a day
You are allergic to the sun	Histaminum 5 CH 2 pillules 3 times a day *combined with* Muriaticum acidum 5 CH 2 pillules 3 times a day

See also: Burns, page 97.

ADVICE

Excessive exposure to the sun is dangerous to the skin and may cause cancer. But who can resist the feeling of happiness from the warm sensation of sunbathing on a sandy beach? Take advantage of this, but in moderation and with common sense. Cover yourself well with high-protection sunscreen, especially by the sea or in the mountains, where the reflection of the sun's rays makes them stronger. Choose to expose your skin at less dangerous times and absolutely avoid 11 a.m.–4 p.m. Comprehensively protect children, especially very young children: hat, T-shirt, sunglasses, and sunscreen on parts that are still exposed. Our children's skin is even more fragile than our own.

WHIPLASH

See: Blow, shock, trauma, page 120.

CUTS

Skin cuts due to a sharp object (such as a knife, scissors, lancet in a surgical operation). The cut is painful and the wound bleeds.

INDICATIONS	TREATMENT
For all types of cuts	Arnica montana 9 CH 2 pillules 3 times a day *combined with* Staphysagria 5 CH 2 pillules 3 times a day
Local application	Calendula mother tincture *and* Echinacea mother tincture *and* Centella asiatica mother tincture on sterile compresses

ADVICE

If the cut is large, have it stitched up or use several steri-strips.

MUSCLE PAIN AND STIFFNESS

Muscle pain is similar to stiff muscles. The pain most often occurs after physical effort that you are unaccustomed to (for example, taking up a sport again after a long break) or after an illness.

INDICATIONS	TREATMENT
The pain is due to physical effort and your muscles are painful	Arnica montana 9 CH 2 pillules 3 times a day
The pain is due to physical effort; your muscles, bones, and eyes are painful	Arnica montana 9 CH 2 pillules 3 times a day *combined with* Eupatorium perfoliatum 5 CH 2 pillules 3 times a day
The pain is due to an illness (like the flu), and you are worn out	Gelsemium 5 CH 2 pillules 3 times a day
The soreness causes a pain that is like a spasm or cramp	Sarcolacticum acidum 5 CH 2 pillules 3 times a day
The soreness is less painful at rest and when compressed by a bandage	Bryonia 5 CH 2 pillules 3 times a day
The soreness is less painful when you move	Rhus toxicodendron 5 CH 2 pillules 3 times a day

ADVICE

Always remember to warm up before starting physical activity: run in place, stretch, and move each part of your body gently for a few moments.

If you feel pain, you should only think about recovering: drink sweet fruit juice and eat carbohydrates (such as bread or pasta) slowly; relax if you can; have a massage; arrange for a sauna session (except if you have had renal colic or deficient venous circulation); and do not hesitate to let yourself take a nap.

CRAMPS

Violent contraction, painful, involuntary, and temporary, of one or more muscles. Cramps are due to buildup of lactic acid in the muscle, naturally produced when you make an effort. They are often seen in people who do a lot of physical activity.

INDICATIONS	TREATMENT
The cramp is in a muscle	Cuprum metallicum 5 CH 2 pillules 3 times a day
The cramp is abdominal, and it is less painful when you bend over	Magnesia phosphorica 5 CH 2 pillules 3 times a day
The abdominal cramp is caused by an emotion (such as indignation or fear), and it is less painful with pressure	Colocynthis 5 CH 2 pillules 3 times a day
You have cramps when you get your period; physical pain alternates with mental/emotional problems	Actaea racemosa 5 CH 2 pillules 3 times a day
Your cramps are due to compression of the arteries and circulatory problems	Secale cornutum 5 CH 2 pillules 3 times a day

ADVICE

To get rid of cramps rapidly, massage and stretch the muscle. The movement may hurt, but it will help to eliminate the lactic acid buildup responsible for the pain.

FISSURE

Crack in the skin, deep or otherwise, generally situated at the corners of the mouth, on the hands, the feet, or on the breasts, especially when breastfeeding.

INDICATIONS	TREATMENT
The fissure has a honey-like discharge, which can form crusts; your skin is dry, and you do not sweat	Graphites 5 CH 2 pillules 3 times a day
The fissure, of blackish appearance, appears especially in winter	Petroleum 5 CH 2 pillules 3 times a day
The fissure is situated on the breast (during breastfeeding, for example) and your skin is dry	Graphites 5 CH 2 pillules 3 times a day *combined with* Castor equi 4 CH Local application of ointment

ADVICE

Avoid ointment and dressings that soak the skin and generally anything that could keep the fissure in a damp environment. Rather, ensure that the skin remains dry, and use internal treatments that work better for these kinds of symptoms.

INDIGESTION, LIVER PROBLEMS

See: Indigestion after excessive eating, page 200.

CYSTITIS, URINARY TRACT INFECTION

Inflammation of the bladder and the urinary tract. You suffer from a burning sensation and pain when you urinate and have a continual desire to pass urine, although there may not be very much.

INDICATIONS	TREATMENT
You have a renal calculus (you pass urine easily when standing, but it is impossible for you to do so when sitting)	Formica rufa 5 CH 2 pillules 3 times a day *combined with* Sarsaparilla 5 CH 2 pillules 3 times a day *and with* Bladder 4 CH 2 pillules 3 times a day
You have a constant desire to urinate	Lilium tigrinum 5 CH 2 pillules 3 times a day
There is urinary irritation or burning on urinating, with blood in the urine	Cantharis 5 CH 2 pillules 3 times a day *combined with* Mercurius corrosivus 5 CH 2 pillules 3 times a day
Your urine smells bad	Benzoicum acidum 5 CH 2 pillules 3 times a day
You have difficulty urinating; you suffer from edema	Apis mellifica 5 CH 2 pillules 3 times a day
You have spasms in the groin area, with calculi	Pareira brava 5 CH 2 pillules 3 times a day
The cystitis causes burning and fever	Belladonna 5 CH 2 pillules 3 times a day

INDICATIONS	TREATMENT
The cystitis gives rise to burning sensations, which are even stronger between 1 and 3 a.m. and you feel better when heat is applied	Arsenicum album 5 CH 2 pillules 3 times a day
The cystitis follows sexual contact	Staphysagria 5 CH 2 pillules 3 times a day
You have repeated urinary tract infections	Colibacillinum 4 CH (*Bacillus coli*) 2 pillules 3 times a day *or* Serum anticolibacillaire 5 CH 2 pillules 3 times a day
You have repeated urinary tract infections and a tendency to depression	Sepia 9 CH 2 pillules 3 times a day
You have hypertrophy of the prostate, accompanied by spasms and difficulty urinating	Sabal serrulata 5 CH 2 pillules 3 times a day

ADVICE

Cystitis is mainly a women's problem and is due to bacteria that are present in the intestines or in the anal area.

- Drink a lot of water every day to "flush" the bladder.
- Get medical advice early, to avoid developing a kidney infection.

Be careful with the hygiene of your intimate areas. After using the toilet, do not clean yourself from the back toward the front but from the front toward the back, to keep the bacteria away from the urethra.

TORN MUSCLE

Muscle condition accompanied by sudden pain. All movements of this muscle immediately become very painful. There is sometimes slight edema.

INDICATIONS	TREATMENT
In all cases	Arnica montana 9 CH 2 pillules 3 times a day
To soothe the muscle	Sarcolacticum acidum 5 CH 2 pillules 3 times a day
The tear is accompanied by muscle cramps	Cuprum metallicum 5 CH 2 pillules 3 times a day
The pain improves with cold or application of ice	Ledum palustre 5 CH 2 pillules 3 times a day
The tear is accompanied by edema, it feels better when cold compresses are applied	Apis mellifica 5 CH 2 pillules 3 times a day

ADVICE

To avoid muscle problems, especially before physical activity, give preference to foods rich in complex sugars, fiber, and magnesium and remember to drink a lot of liquids. A healthy lifestyle is the bottom line. And do not forget to warm up!

ITCHING, PRURITUS

It feels hot, you scratch, it stings, it tickles—in short, it irritates you and you cannot leave it alone.

INDICATIONS	TREATMENT
The itching is aggravated by water and by heat (of the bed, for example) but helped by cold	Sulfur 5 CH 2 pillules 3 times a day
The irritated area is like urticaria, with small blisters	Urtica urens 5 CH 2 pillules 3 times a day *or* Dolichos pruriens 5 CH 2 pillules 3 times a day
The irritated area is covered with small blisters seeping with a whitish liquid	Mezereum 5 CH 2 pillules 3 times a day
There is slight edema and burning; the itching is helped by cold compresses	Apis mellifica 5 CH 2 pillules 3 times a day
The skin is hot, burning, and dry	Belladonna 5 CH 2 pillules 3 times a day
The itching is due to an allergy (for example, costume jewelry or laundry detergent)	Histaminum 5 CH 2 pillules 3 times a day *or* Isotherapic of the allergen 5 CH 2 pillules 3 times a day

INDICATIONS	TREATMENT
The itching is due to a food allergy; it weeps if you scratch it, and you feel sleepy	Phenobarbital 5 CH 2 pillules 3 times a day
The itching is due to eczema on unhealthy skin; it is worse with water or heat (of the bed, for example); you are chilly	Psorinum 9 CH 2 pillules 3 times a day
The itching is due to dry eczema and better with a hot water bottle; you are chilly, but the fresh air makes you feel better	Arsenicum album 9 CH 2 pillules 3 times a day
The eczema is oozing	Graphites 5 CH 2 pillules 3 times a day
The eczema is a winter eczema with fissures	Petroleum 5 CH 2 pillules 3 times a day
The itching comes on when you undress	Rumex crispus 5 CH 2 pillules 3 times a day
The itching is due to worms (especially in the anus and the nose)	Cina 5 CH 2 pillules 3 times a day
The itching comes on after radiation therapy or exposure to X-rays	Radium bromatum 5 CH 2 pillules 3 times a day

INDICATIONS	TREATMENT
The itching affects the genital organs	Sulfur 5 CH 2 pillules 3 times a day *or* Lilium tigrinum 5 CH 2 pillules 3 times a day
The itching causes sexual hypersensitivity	Platina 9 CH 2 pillules 3 times a day

ADVICE

People of the psoric type are very prone to itching. The more you scratch, the more it itches. Take anything that helps you—cold compresses, hot baths, cool breezes—and avoid contact with clothing or jewelry while waiting for the remedies to have an effect.

DERMATOSIS OF HANDS AND FEET

Skin condition that often takes the form of slight eczema accompanied by itching.

INDICATIONS	TREATMENT
The eczema is confined to the hands and the soles of the feet, with small blisters	Anagallis arvensis 5 CH 2 pillules 3 times a day
The eczema is accompanied by edema	Bovista 5 CH 2 pillules 3 times a day

INDICATIONS	TREATMENT
When there is fungus	Candida albicans 5 CH *combined with* Complex remedy with Lappa major 4 CH and Viola tricolor 4 CH *(See: Complex remedies, page 320).* 2 pillules 3 times a day
Local application	Bellis perennis mother tincture Calendula mother tincture Centella asiatica mother tincture Mimosa tenuiflora mother tincture

See also: Itching, pruritus, page 130; Eczema, page 147.

ADVICE

On the hands, in particular, skin conditions can be due to allergies. Avoid costume jewelry and nickel and choose metals you are less likely to have a reaction to (gold, silver). Other products, such as cosmetics or home cleaning products, may also cause contact dermatitis.

If you are susceptible to these reactions, wear gloves as often as possible to protect yourself. And, where there is an allergy, consider having an isotherapic remedy prepared from the substance responsible. (See: Isotherapy, page 64.)

DIABETES

Metabolic disorder leading to an abnormal presence of sugar in the blood. There are two types of diabetes: insulin-dependent diabetes, when the pancreas cannot produce insulin, and non-insulin-dependent diabetes, when the pancreas still functions but is not sufficiently effective. In the second instance, you can stimulate the pancreas to help it to create its own insulin, in different ways.

INDICATIONS	TREATMENT
Phytotherapy	Allium cepa mother tincture 30 drops 3 times a day *combined with* Eucalyptus mother tincture 30 drops 3 times a day *and also* Juglans regia mother tincture 30 drops 3 times a day
Organ support therapy	*To stimulate the pancreas* Pancreas 4 CH 2 pillules 3 times a day *or to stimulate the production of insulin* Insulinum 4 CH 2 pillules 3 times a day
You have adult-onset diabetes, are overweight, and you like sugary foods	Sulfur 5 CH 2 pillules 3 times a day
You have diabetes and are not overweight; you like sugary foods and chocolate; you are hyperactive	Argentum nitricum 5 CH 2 pillules 3 times a day
You have a hyperthyroid condition and are anxious and agitated	Arsenicum iodatum 5 CH 2 pillules 3 times a day

INDICATIONS	TREATMENT
You have a hyperthyroid condition and are very thin, agitated, and always hot	Iodum 5 CH 2 pillules 3 times a day *combined with* Thyroid 15 CH 2 pillules 3 times a day

ADVICE

To treat diabetes correctly with homeopathy, you should treat the patient as a whole. The remedy for the diabetic person is more important than the treatment of diabetes itself. Nux vomica will suit a stressed CEO; Lachesis, a voluble person with alcoholic tendencies; and Sulfur, a person who likes eating and drinking, is always hot, and craves sweet foods. There can be as many remedies as people who are ill. It is essential to seek advice from a homeopathic doctor.

DIARRHEA

Liquid stool, abundant and very frequent. You have abdominal pain and rush to the toilet many times a day. The diarrhea may have numerous causes: gastroenteritis, indigestion, too much unripe fruit, infection, traveling, medications, and even sometimes emotions or stress.

INDICATIONS	TREATMENT
In all cases, and especially if you do not feel better after a bowel movement; you also have nausea; your tongue remains pink	Ipecac 5 CH 2 pillules 3 times a day

INDICATIONS	TREATMENT
The diarrhea causes intense and prolonged fatigue	China rubra 7 CH 2 pillules 3 times a day
You have liver problems, you are tired, you feel worse in the evening, and your stools are gushing	Phosphorus 5 CH 2 pillules 3 times a day
Your diarrhea is abundant, liquid, and gushing	Podophyllum peltatum 5 CH 2 pillules 3 times a day
Your diarrhea is painless but abundant and dehydrating	Ricinus communis 5 CH (Castor oil) 2 pillules 3 times a day
The diarrhea is bloody and you have amebiasis	Mercurius corrosivus 5 CH 2 pillules 3 times a day *combined with* Ipecac 5 CH 2 pillules 3 times a day
The diarrhea contains greenish mucus	Mercurius solubilis 5 CH 2 pillules 3 times a day *combined with* Ipecac 5 CH 2 pillules 3 times a day
The diarrhea is accompanied by irritation of the intestines	Senna 5 CH 2 pillules 3 times a day
The diarrhea is due to indigestion and accompanied by nausea	Antimonium crudum 5 CH 2 pillules 3 times a day

INDICATIONS	TREATMENT
The diarrhea is due to food poisoning; it is accompanied by nausea and abdominal pain; better with a hot water bottle	Arsenicum album 5 CH 2 pillules 3 times a day
You are agitated and anxious; you feel worse between 1 a.m. and 3 a.m. and feel cold, but better with fresh air	Arsenicum album 15 CH 2 pillules 3 times a day
The diarrhea is resistant to all treatment	Paratyphoidinum B 9 CH 2 pillules 3 times a day
The diarrhea is accompanied by delirium	Baptisia tinctoria 5 CH 2 pillules 3 times a day
The diarrhea is accompanied by cold sweats and malaise, even fainting	Veratrum album 5 CH 2 pillules 3 times a day
You also have hemorrhoids and your sphincters are a bit weak, allowing small quantities of stool to escape	Aloe 5 CH 2 pillules 3 times a day
You have eaten unripe fruits	Rheum 5 CH 2 pillules 3 times a day
Your baby has greenish diarrhea due to teething and is very agitated	Chamomilla 15 CH 2 pillules 3 times a day

INDICATIONS	TREATMENT
The diarrhea is due to stage fright; you are nervous and agitated	Argentum nitricum 5 CH 2 pillules 3 times a day
The diarrhea is due to stage fright; you go to pieces	Gelsemium 9 CH 2 pillules 3 times a day
The diarrhea is due to lactose intolerance	Aethusa cynapium 5 CH 2 pillules 3 times a day
The diarrhea is accompanied by spasms	Magnesia carbonica 5 CH 2 pillules 3 times a day *or* Magnesia phosphorica 5 CH 2 pillules 3 times a day

ADVICE

You should be aware that profuse diarrhea entails a loss of fluids and electrolytes and may cause dehydration. This can be serious in babies or the elderly, so it is necessary to monitor their weight carefully and make sure that they drink regularly, even if—and especially if—they are not thirsty.

PAIN

Painful sensation felt in one part of the body, with greater or lesser intensity, more or less regularly occurring and corresponding to a condition, illness, or traumatic event.

For each pain, whatever the location, the homeopath will seek to help the person who is suffering before focusing their interest on the pain itself.

INDICATIONS	TREATMENT
The pain is helped by cold and ice	Ledum palustre 5 CH 2 pillules 3 times a day
The pain is helped by cold and accompanied by edema	Apis mellifica 5 CH 2 pillules 3 times a day
The pain is helped by heat to the local area	Arsenicum album 5 CH 2 pillules 3 times a day
The pain, often at night, is aggravated by cold and by heat	Mercurius solubilis 5 CH 2 pillules 3 times a day
The pain, aggravated by humid heat, is even more intense at night	Rhododendron 5 CH 2 pillules 3 times a day
The pain is triggered by sudden dry cold	Aconitum napellus 5 CH 2 pillules 3 times a day
The pain is triggered by humidity (rain) or being near to a source of humidity (lake, ocean)	Dulcamara 5 CH 2 pillules 3 times a day
The pain is helped by movement and aggravated by humid cold	Rhus toxicodendron 5 CH 2 pillules 3 times a day
The pain is helped by slow movement	Pulsatilla 5 CH 2 pillules 3 times a day
The pain is helped by rapid, even brisk, movement	Sepia 5 CH 2 pillules 3 times a day
The pain is worse when you stay still	Valeriana 5 CH 2 pillules 3 times a day

INDICATIONS	TREATMENT
The pain resembles a bruise, a stiff muscle, or muscle soreness; it is better with rest, but even a bed seems too hard	Arnica montana 9 CH 2 pillules 3 times a day
The pain is better with rest and pressure	Bryonia 5 CH 2 pillules 3 times a day
The pain is better when you are resting; you feel worn out, both physically and mentally	Gelsemium 9 CH 2 pillules 3 times a day
The pain is better when you are distracted or aggravated by the presence of someone you do not like and changes according to your mood	Ignatia amara 9 CH 2 pillules 3 times a day
The pain is accompanied by fever and redness	Belladonna 5 CH 2 pillules 3 times a day
The pain is accompanied by edema	Apis mellifica 5 CH 2 pillules 3 times a day
You suffer in silence; you are stoic	Natrum muriaticum 9 CH 2 pillules 3 times a day or Sepia 9 CH 2 pillules 3 times a day
You shout with pain; you are sensitive to noise and light	Nux vomica 9 CH 2 pillules 3 times a day

INDICATIONS	TREATMENT
You are hypersensitive to the pain itself; it makes you aggressive	Chamomilla 9 CH 2 pillules 3 times a day
You are irritable at night; you do not feel it during the day, but you are worn out	Opium 9 CH 2 pillules 3 times a day

ADVICE

After analyzing your behavior and choosing your remedy according to what triggers the pain, you can combine it with a remedy to act more specifically on the exact type of pain (see the following). It is also important to know the location (left or right) of the pain and even the time of aggravation; both are useful indicators for choosing the most effective treatment.

PAIN—JOINTS

INDICATIONS	TREATMENT
For pain in the small joints and possibly attacks of gout	Colchicum 5 CH 2 pillules 3 times a day *combined with* Caulophyllum 5 CH 2 pillules 3 times a day
For pain in the fingers and rheumatism of the phalanges aggravated by humidity	Actaea spicata 5 CH 2 pillules 3 times a day

INDICATIONS	TREATMENT
If there is inflammation	Guaiacum 5 CH 2 pillules 3 times a day
The pain is due to the presence of uric acid	Uricum acidum 5 CH 2 pillules 3 times a day *combined with* Colchicum 5 CH 2 pillules 3 times a day

See also: Osteoarthritis, page 82; Sprains, page 154.

PAIN—TEETH

INDICATIONS	TREATMENT
In all cases	Calcarea fluorica 5 CH 2 pillules 3 times a day
In the case of teething in a baby, ameliorated by rocking or passive movement and often accompanied by greenish diarrhea	Chamomilla 9 CH 2 pillules 3 times a day
The teeth are hypersensitive to cold and heat	Hypericum perforatum 5 CH 2 pillules 3 times a day
Your teeth are fragile, blackish	Kreosotum 5 CH 2 pillules 3 times a day

See also: Cavities, page 100.

PAIN—BACK

INDICATIONS	TREATMENT
Your profession causes back pain (for example, a dentist bending forward all day long)	Arnica montana 9 CH 2 pillules 3 times a day *combined with* Kalium phosphoricum 5 CH 2 pillules 3 times a day
Your back pain alternates with mental/emotional symptoms	Actaea racemosa 5 CH 2 pillules 3 times a day
The pain is worse at dusk	Phosphorus 5 CH 2 pillules 3 times a day
Your pain is due to demineralization, and your extremities are cold	Silicea 5 CH 2 pillules 3 times a day

See also: Low back pain, page 211.

PAIN—LUMBAR

INDICATIONS	TREATMENT
The pain is better when you stretch out	Dioscorea villosa 5 CH 2 pillules 3 times a day
The pain is better when you bend over	Magnesia phosphorica 5 CH 2 pillules 3 times a day

See also: Pain—back.

PAIN—LIMBS

INDICATIONS	TREATMENT
The pain is accompanied by incessant restless movement	Zincum metallicum 5 CH 2 pillules 3 times a day
The pain is accompanied by stiffening of the limbs	Plumbum 5 CH 2 pillules 3 times a day
The pain is accompanied by trembling	Gelsemium 5 CH 2 pillules 3 times a day

PAIN—MUSCLE

See also: Muscle pain and stiffness, page 123; Torn muscle, page 129; Pulled muscle, page 150.

PAIN—BONES

INDICATIONS	TREATMENT
The pain is in the outer part of the bone	Aurum metallicum 5 CH 2 pillules 3 times a day
The bone pain is generalized, you have sore muscles	Eupatorium perfoliatum 5 CH 2 pillules 3 times a day
The pain is more intense at night	Syphilinum 5 CH 2 pillules 3 times a day
Growing pains	Phosphoricum acidum 5 CH 2 pillules 3 times a day

INDICATIONS	TREATMENT
To accelerate bone building after a traumatic injury or in osteoporosis	Symphytum 5 CH 2 pillules 3 times a day

See also: Fractures, page 170.

PAIN—BREAST

INDICATIONS	TREATMENT
If there is a hematoma	Arnica montana 9 CH 2 pillules 3 times a day
The pain is localized in the soft parts	Bellis perennis 5 CH 2 pillules 3 times a day

See also: Breastfeeding, page 59.

PAIN—TENDONS

INDICATIONS	TREATMENT
In all cases	Ruta graveolens 5 CH 2 pillules 3 times a day *combined with* Arnica montana 9 CH 2 pillules 3 times a day
The pain is better when you move	*Add* Rhus toxicidendron 5 CH 2 pillules 3 times a day

ABRASION

Superficial wound to the skin, like a scratch.

INDICATIONS	TREATMENT
In all cases	Pyrogenium 9 CH 2 pillules 3 times a day
You have been scratched by a sharp object (such as a knife, razor blade, sheet of paper)	*Add* Staphysagria 5 CH 2 pillules 3 times a day
You have been pricked with a needle or by the thorn of a rose	*Add* Silicea 5 CH 2 pillules 3 times a day *combined with* Hypericum perforatum 5 CH 2 pillules 3 times a day
The abrasion takes the form of small, yellowish fissures	*Add* Nitricum acidum 5 CH 2 pillules 3 times a day
The abrasion has begun to ulcerate	*Add* Argentum nitricum 5 CH 2 pillules 3 times a day *or* Kalium bichromicum 5 CH 2 pillules 3 times a day

ADVICE

Always begin by cleaning the wound using a compress soaked with Calendula mother tincture. If you regularly work in the garden, consider updating your tetanus vaccination.

CORYZA, NASAL DISCHARGE

See: Coryza, rhinitis, colds, page 117.

ECZEMA

Skin condition recognizable by the appearance of small vesicles distributed in red patches. The eczema develops in flare-ups. It can be atopic (resulting from a generalized allergic state), from contact (reaction to a product that causes allergies, such as nickel, chrome, flowers, cosmetics, and so on), or varicose (a complication of venous insufficiency). It can appear in different forms: with vesicles, weeping or dry, with patches of skin that become detached, or flaking of skin.

INDICATIONS	TREATMENT
The eczema is dry, with burning sensations better with local heat (warm compress or hot water bottle)	Arsenicum album 5 CH 2 pillules 3 times a day
The eczema is dry with itching; your skin flakes	Berberis vulgaris 5 CH 2 pillules 3 times a day
The eczema is dry and aggravated at the beach	Natrum muriaticum 5 CH 2 pillules 3 times a day
The eczema is dry; your skin is yellow and wrinkled	Sepia 5 CH 2 pillules 3 times a day
The eczema weeps slightly, forming crusts when it dries; you are chilly and do not heal well	Graphites 5 CH 2 pillules 3 times a day

INDICATIONS	TREATMENT
The eczema is weeping and infected	Staphylococcinum 5 CH 2 pillules 3 times a day
The winter eczema is painful and has black fissures	Petroleum 5 CH 2 pillules 3 times a day
The eczema is located in the genital area	Lilium tigrinum 5 CH 2 pillules 3 times a day
The eczema is located in the genital area and is accompanied by extreme itching and burning, with vesicles; it alternates with diarrhea	Croton tiglium 5 CH 2 pillules 3 times a day
The eczema is in the auditory canal	Calcarea picrata 5 CH 2 pillules 3 times a day
The eczema is on the hands	Actaea spicata 5 CH 2 pillules 3 times a day
The eczema is on the scalp and the face, accompanied by itching	Staphysagria 5 CH 2 pillules 3 times a day
You are congestive; you have red extremities (ears, lips, and so on)	Drainage remedy (of the liver, the kidney and the skin) *(See: Complex remedies, page 320)* 20 drops 3 times a day *then* Sulfur 5 CH 2 pillules 3 times a day
You have a rounded build	Calcarea carbonicum 9 CH 1 dose a week

INDICATIONS	TREATMENT
You are chilly, your eczema is aggravated by water and heat, and it appears after a parasitic disease or a sexually transmitted disease	Psorinum 5 CH 2 pillules 3 times a day
Your eczema is better when you eat	Anacardium orientale 5 CH 2 pillules 3 times a day
VARICOSE ECZEMA	
The eczema is varicose and aggravated by heat	Sulfur 5 CH 2 pillules 3 times a day
The eczema is varicose and ameliorated by local heat	Arsenicum album 5 CH 2 pillules 3 times a day

ADVICE

In the case of eczema, the homeopathic doctor will be especially interested in the whole person who is ill: their body shape, their behavior, the state of their skin. It is sometimes difficult to properly identify eczema and its cause: allergic terrain or one-off reaction, purely physical phenomena or manifestation of stress. It is preferable to consult a specialist before selecting the right remedy.

PREMATURE EJACULATION

Premature emission of sperm, before consummation of the sexual act, or too rapidly after penetration.

INDICATIONS	TREATMENT
You are agitated and nervous; you want to finish before you have started	Argentum nitricum 9 CH 2 pillules 3 times a day

ADVICE

A psychological approach to this problem may be indispensable to help the man to concentrate on all aspects of sexual contact other than coitus: foreplay, caresses, massage. A one-off technique called pressure sometimes has good results: at the moment the man feels that he is going to ejaculate, press the base of the penis between two fingers for a few seconds. This simple technique can delay the orgasm without affecting the erection.

PULLED MUSCLE

Accidental and painful traction exercised on a muscle.

INDICATIONS	TREATMENT
In all cases	Arnica montana 9 CH 2 pillules 3 times a day *combined with* Cuprum metallicum 5 CH 2 pillules 3 times a day *and* Lacticum acidum 5 CH 2 pillules 3 times a day *and* Magnesia phosphorica 5 CH 2 pillules 3 times a day

INDICATIONS	TREATMENT
The tendons are painful	Ruta graveolens 5 CH 2 pillules 3 times a day
The pain is helped by the application of ice	Ledum palustre 5 CH 2 pillules 3 times a day

ADVICE

After the trauma responsible for the pulled muscle, immediately apply an icepack to the painful part for at least 15 minutes. This will help the pain and improve the action of the remedies.

EMOTIONALISM, HYPERSENSITIVITY

Tendency to feel intense emotions to an unreasonable extent, sometimes leading to a loss of self-control. The emotions are expressed in different ways: mental/emotional (fear, joy, weeping, anger, grief) or physical (trembling, palpitations, sweating, urge to use the toilet, clammy hands, redness). The causes are varied: love, stress, anxiety, surprise, failure, joy, and so on.

INDICATIONS	TREATMENT
For disappointed love	Ignatia amara 7 CH 2 pillules 3 times a day
For paradoxical manifestations of emotion (you laugh during a funeral, you cry at a baptism)	Ignatia amara 7 CH 2 pillules 3 times a day
For extreme joy (winning a bet, success on an exam)	Coffea cruda 7 CH 2 pillules 3 times a day

INDICATIONS	TREATMENT
For great emotional pain (bereavement, failure)	Arnica montana 9 CH 2 pillules 3 times a day *combined with* Gelsemium 9 CH 2 pillules 3 times a day
For psychological shock	Arnica montana 15 CH 2 pillules 3 times a day
For emotions that paralyze, when you are unable to react	Gelsemium 15 CH 2 pillules 3 times a day
For emotions that excite, when you are unable to stay in one place	Argentum nitricum 7 CH 2 pillules 3 times a day
For emotions that give rise to incessant movement of the legs	Zincum metallicum 7 CH 2 pillules 3 times a day
For emotions that give rise to incessant movement of the hands	Kalium bromatum 7 CH 2 pillules 3 times a day
For people who are timid, who cry often, and feel tired, even depressed	Ambra grisea 7 CH 2 pillules 3 times a day
For public displays of emotion, causing you uneasiness and theatrical reactions	Moschus 5 CH 2 pillules 3 times a day
You are hypersensitive and you alternate between moments of agitation and somnolence	Valeriana 5 CH 2 pillules 3 times a day

ADVICE

To attempt to control your emotional reactions, you can try to prepare yourself for upcoming events. Anticipating stressful situations sometimes helps to control them. Techniques such as yoga or relaxation are also a great help.

TONSILLITIS

See: Sore throat, tonsillitis, throat pain, pharyngitis, page 67.

BREAST ENGORGEMENT

See: Breastfeeding, page 59.

HOARSENESS, APHONIA

Change in the timbre of the voice, sometimes leading to losing it completely, aphonia.

INDICATIONS	TREATMENT
You are hoarse because you have been speaking for too long	Arnica montana 9 CH 2 pillules 3 times a day
You are hoarse in the morning, and cold drinks help your voice	Causticum 7 CH 2 pillules 3 times a day
You are hoarse on waking, but your voice comes back when you speak	Rhus toxicodendron 5 CH 2 pillules 3 times a day
You are hoarse in the evening	Phosphorus 7 CH 2 pillules 3 times a day

INDICATIONS	TREATMENT
You go from low to high without being able to control your voice	Arum triphyllum 5 CH 2 pillules 3 times a day
You are drastically hoarse after exposure to a draft or dry cold	Aconitum napellus 5 CH 2 pillules 3 times a day
You are drastically hoarse after exposure to a draft or damp cold	Dulcamara 5 CH 2 pillules 3 times a day
You have a very husky voice due to cold and damp in the morning	Manganum metallicum 5 CH 2 pillules 3 times a day

ADVICE

Just as with muscles, the vocal cords may need warming up and may get tired when they work. Before you sing or go to a game and yell to support your favorite team, do some vocal or vocalizing exercises. Allow yourself short pauses to recuperate, and consider taking a bottle of cool water with you. A drink of water from time to time always helps.

SPRAINS

Sudden, painful lesion in a ligament or a joint, due to a traumatic injury (often a twist) and accompanied by edema. The classic situation is that you twist your ankle by missing a step on the staircase or injure your knee when you fall while skiing. You hear a crack, your joint swells up, and you feel pain.

INDICATIONS	TREATMENT
To treat the traumatic injury	*Take, as soon as possible* Arnica montana 9 CH 2 pillules 3 times a day
The tendons are affected	Arnica montana 9 CH 2 pillules 3 times a day *combined with* Ruta graveolens 5 CH 2 pillules 3 times a day
You suffer from weakening of the joints or ligaments	Natrum carbonicum 5 CH 2 pillules 3 times a day
The pain is better with rest and pressure from a bandage	Arnica montana 9 CH 2 pillules 3 times a day *combined with* Bryonia 5 CH 2 pillules 3 times a day
The pain is helped by movement	Arnica montana 9 CH 2 pillules 3 times a day *combined with* Rhus toxicodendron 5 CH 2 pillules 3 times a day
The pain improves with cold or application of ice	Arnica montana 9 CH 2 pillules 3 times a day *combined with* Ledum palustre 5 CH 2 pillules 3 times a day

INDICATIONS	TREATMENT
The inflammation and edema are better with cold compresses	Arnica montana 9 CH 2 pillules 3 times a day *combined with* Apis mellifica 5 CH 2 pillules 3 times a day
In the case of repeated sprains	Calcarea fluorica 9 CH 2 pillules 3 times a day

ADVICE

Do not dismiss a sprain as unimportant: if it is not properly treated, it can cause a problem or even disability in the long term. Good treatment and rest, sometimes even immobilization, are essential.

INCONTINENCE, BEDWETTING (ENURESIS)

Urinary incontinence, usually at night in children (it may not necessarily wake them) or in elderly people who are beginning to lose awareness of their body.

INDICATIONS	TREATMENT
IN CHILDREN	
The child begins to wet the bed after a physical trauma	Arnica montana 9 CH 2 pillules 3 times a day
The child begins to wet the bed after a blow to the head or a fall	Arnica montana 9 CH 2 pillules 3 times a day *combined with* Natrum sulphuricum 9 CH 2 pillules 3 times a day

INDICATIONS	TREATMENT
The child begins to wet the bed after a shock; the child is very anxious and trembling	Arnica montana 9 CH 2 pillules 3 times a day *combined with* Gelsemium 9 CH 2 pillules 3 times a day
The child wets the bed after anesthesia	Arnica montana 9 CH 2 pillules 3 times a day *combined with* Opium 5 CH 2 pillules 3 times a day
The child wets the bed from distraction	Ignatia amara 9 CH 2 pillules 3 times a day
The child wets the bed from a desire for attention	Pulsatilla 9 CH 2 pillules 3 times a day
The child wets the bed because of something he can't express (for example, jealousy at the birth of a younger brother, lack of love)	Staphysagria 9 CH 2 pillules 3 times a day
The child does not wake when he wets the bed	Opium 5 CH 2 pillules 3 times a day *combined with* Causticum 9 CH 2 pillules 3 times a day
IN AN ELDERLY PERSON	
In case of weakening of the bladder or the urethra	Sepia 9 CH 2 pillules 3 times a day

INDICATIONS	TREATMENT
In case of prolapsed organs	Calcarea fluorica 9 CH 2 pillules 3 times a day
In case of leakage when you cough, when you laugh, or when you make an effort to do something	Causticum 5 CH 2 pillules 3 times a day

ADVICE

Do not blame the child: enuresis is often just a way of expressing themselves. There is no "right" age to stop wetting the bed, and the child is not necessarily aware of it happening. Try to discuss it with them to find the cause of their annoying problem, and do not hesitate to consult a psychologist.

BURPING

See: Flatulence (eructations, burps), bloating, page 56.

SNEEZING

Sudden, noisy exhalation from the nose and the mouth due to irritation of the mucous membranes of the nose. Bless you!

INDICATIONS	TREATMENT
You have bouts of sneezing	Sabadilla 5 CH 2 pillules 3 times a day
The wings of the nostrils are irritated, and the sneezing is accompanied by a liquid, watery discharge	Allium cepa 5 CH 2 pillules 3 times a day

INDICATIONS	TREATMENT
The eyes burn, and the sneezing is accompanied by a liquid, watery discharge	Euphrasia 5 CH 2 pillules 3 times a day
The eyes and the nose are irritated	Naphtalinum 5 CH 2 pillules 3 times a day

See also: Coryza, rhinitis, colds, page 117; Allergies, page 61.

ADVICE

Avoid allopathic medicines intended to prevent sneezing. Decongestive products often have side effects (somnolence, and so on). To clean the nose, use saline solution. A sneeze is emunctory (eliminates waste from the body); it is essential not to stop it.

EXCITATION, HYPERACTIVITY

State of agitation and irritation. You cannot stay still; you feel impatient, in a hurry, and sometimes irritable.

INDICATIONS	TREATMENT
IN ALL CASES	
The excitement is accompanied by vertigo	Argentum nitricum 9 CH 2 pillules 3 times a day
The excitation comes on especially at night, but during the day you are calm, even sluggish	Opium 9 CH 2 pillules 3 times a day
You are excited by a rush of ideas or after good news	Coffea cruda 9 CH 2 pillules 3 times a day

INDICATIONS	TREATMENT
The excitement is manifested by restless legs	Zincum metallicum 9 CH 2 pillules 3 times a day
The excitement shows up as restlessness in the hands	Kalium bromatum 9 CH 2 pillules 3 times a day
You need to walk slowly in the open air	Pulsatilla 9 CH 2 pillules 3 times a day
You need to walk quickly	Sepia 9 CH 2 pillules 3 times a day
You feel calmer when you are moving	Rhus toxicodendron 9 CH 2 pillules 3 times a day
You talk a great deal, without stopping, then you go into a state of depression, aggravated by alcohol	Lachesis 9 CH 2 pillules 3 times a day
WHEN IT IS A CHILD	
The child is agitated, aggressive, cannot sleep without light	Stramonium 9 CH 2 pillules 3 times a day
The child touches everything they can reach and cannot stay still	Tarentula hispana 9 CH 2 pillules 3 times a day
The excitation is calmed by passive movement (like rocking for a baby) and intensifies in case of pain	Chamomilla 9 CH 2 pillules 3 times a day

INDICATIONS	TREATMENT
WHEN IT IS AN ELDERLY PERSON	
The elderly person is agitated and exhibitionistic	Hyoscyamus niger 9 CH 2 pillules 3 times a day

ADVICE

You can try to channel the excitation when it gives rise to behavior inappropriate for social life. You could, for example, urge your child to practice a sport based both on combat (as a way to let off steam) and on the execution of movement sequences (promoting self-control), such as judo or karate.

WEAKNESS, FATIGUE, BURNOUT

Lack of physical strength or mental/emotional energy. You feel tired after being ill or following an extreme or prolonged physical effort, or you are overwhelmed by an accumulation of tasks and responsibilities.

INDICATIONS	TREATMENT
You feel physically tired (after moving to a new house or apartment and after physical activity)	Arnica montana 9 CH 2 pillules 3 times a day
Your muscles are tired after expending a considerable physical effort	Lacticum acidum 5 CH 2 pillules 3 times a day
You remain weak after an infectious disease	Natrum muriaticum 9 CH 2 pillules 3 times a day

INDICATIONS	TREATMENT
You are worn out by a high fever; you remain prostrate; you are not thirsty	Gelsemium 9 CH 2 pillules 3 times a day
You feel physically and mentally/emotionally inhibited; your whole body is working in slow motion	Baryta carbonicum 9 CH 2 pillules 3 times a day
You are exhausted and you suddenly collapse, physically and mentally	Gelsemium 9 CH 2 pillules 3 times a day *combined with* Baryta carbonicum 9 CH 2 pillules 3 times a day
You feel weakened by mental work that is too taxing (often an issue for students)	Kalium phosphoricum 9 CH 2 pillules 3 times a day
You are burnt out and you eat snacks to make up for it	Anacardium orientale 9 CH 2 pillules 3 times a day
You feel tired after a loss of body fluids (hemorrhage, diarrhea, nausea, perspiration, repeated ejaculations)	China rubra 5 CH (*Cinchona officinalis*) 2 pillules 3 times a day
You are not sure of yourself, weak, helpless; you feel old before your time	Lycopodium 9 CH 2 pillules 3 times a day
You have venous problems with restless legs	Zincum metallicum 5 CH 2 pillules 3 times a day

INDICATIONS	TREATMENT
You are losing your hair	Selenium 5 CH 2 pillules 3 times a day *combined with* Thallium aceticum 5 CH 2 pillules 3 times a day
You are demineralized	Silicea 9 CH 2 pillules 3 times a day
You have memory lapses	Phosphoricum acidum 9 CH 2 pillules 3 times a day *or* Phosphoricum acidum composite 10 drops 3 times a day
Your tiredness is intense and you become irritable, emotive, manic, and very anxious	Kalium carbonicum 5 CH 2 pillules 3 times a day

See also: Apathy, page 73.

ADVICE

The sensation of tiredness or weakness is a warning sign in your body. Do not underestimate it and do not overestimate yourself! Rest, sleep at regular hours and for long enough, and give yourself breaks: an hour of physical activity in the middle of prolonged mental work (like studying for a test), a ten-minute break every hour when you go on a long hike. The best means of avoiding excessive and disabling tiredness, whether it is physical or mental, is to adopt a healthy lifestyle, keep to moderate levels of effort, and listen to your body. The bottom line is to provide it with a healthy, balanced diet and plenty of water.

EYESTRAIN

Tired eyes with prickling, teariness, heaviness of eyelids, and sometimes vision problems, coming on after intense close work.

INDICATIONS	TREATMENT
In case of overexertion of the eyes	Physostigma 5 CH 2 pillules 3 times a day
You have read or worked on a computer for too long	Arnica montana 9 CH 2 pillules 3 times a day
You have accommodation problems	Ruta graveolens 5 CH 2 pillules 3 times a day
Your eyes are red and tearing	Euphrasia 5 CH 2 pillules 3 times a day
The small blood vessels have burst	Phosphorus tri-iodatus 5 CH 2 pillules 3 times a day
You cannot tolerate light, and your pupils are dilated	Belladonna 5 CH 2 pillules 3 times a day
You cannot tolerate light, and it makes you aggressive	Stramonium 5 CH 2 pillules 3 times a day
You cannot tolerate light, and your eyes are dry	Manganum metallicum 5 CH 2 pillules 3 times a day

ADVICE

If you notice that the small blood vessels in the eye are bursting, contact an ophthalmologist: it could be a case of ocular hypertension. To protect the eyes when you work on a computer, keep to a few simple rules: keep a good distance from the screen (the equivalent of an arm's length); have a break at least every two hours, and use the break to do a few relaxation exercises (ease your head and neck, blink your eyes a few times in succession, yawn); when the tiredness peaks, avoid rubbing your eyes. Even if you think that it helps you, do not put pressure on your eyes: they do not appreciate this at all.

ERYTHEMA OF THE BUTTOCKS, DIAPER RASH IN BABIES

Your baby's buttocks are "on fire": they are red, irritated, and hot.

INDICATIONS	TREATMENT
The erythema is due to being soaked with urine or stool; the baby sleeps on their stomach	Medorrhinum 9 CH 2 pillules 3 times a day (dissolved in the baby's bottle, if need be)
The erythema is due to diarrhea (particularly in the case of teething)	Chamomilla 5 CH 2 pillules 3 times a day (dissolved in the baby's bottle, if need be)
The erythema is due to acid irritation (especially in case of lactose intolerance)	Aethusa cynapium 5 CH 2 pillules 3 times a day (dissolved in the baby's bottle, if need be) combined with Iris versicolor 5 CH 2 pillules 3 times a day (dissolved in the baby's bottle, if need be)
The baby's buttocks are red, hot, and painful	Belladonna 5 CH 2 pillules 3 times a day (dissolved in the baby's bottle, if need be)

ADVICE

Diaper rash in babies can come from an allergy to something in disposable diapers: in this case, try the cotton ones that our grandmothers used. It is vital to treat diarrhea, if present (See: Diarrhea, page 135), and make sure that the baby does not become dehydrated.

FIBROMA, FIBROID

Benign tumor formed out of fibrous tissue, often located in the uterus.

INDICATIONS	TREATMENT
In all cases	Thuja occidentalis 5 CH 2 pillules 3 times a day
Your blood is red	Thuja occidentalis 5 CH 2 pillules 3 times a day *combined with* Sabina 5 CH 2 pillules 3 times a day
Your blood is blackish	Thuja occidentalis 5 CH 2 pillules 3 times a day *combined with* Secale cornutum 5 CH 2 pillules 3 times a day *and with* Ustilago 5 CH 2 pillules 3 times a day
The fibroid is accompanied by a discharge from the reproductive tract	Fraxinus excelsior 5 CH 2 pillules 3 times a day

INDICATIONS	TREATMENT
You also have varicose veins	Hamamelis 5 CH 2 pillules 3 times a day
You have venous congestion in your uterus and pelvis	Aurum muriaticum natronatum 5 CH 2 pillules 3 times a day
You are sad or lonely	Conium 5 CH 2 pillules 3 times a day
You are anemic and asthenic	China rubra 5 CH (*Cinchona officinalis*) 2 pillules 3 times a day

ADVICE

Any tumor, even benign, needs a medical diagnosis, but homeopathy can sometimes preclude the need for an operation.

FEVER

Raised body temperature. Your pulse rate increases, you tremble and have sore muscles, you perspire a lot, you have a burning sensation and stiffness, you are tired, and your mouth is dry.

INDICATIONS	TREATMENT
Burning, "steaming," high fever; you are sweating and cannot tolerate light	Belladonna 5 CH 2 pillules 3 times a day
The fever makes you delirious	Belladonna 15 CH 2 pillules 3 times a day *or* Stramonium 15 CH 2 pillules 3 times a day

INDICATIONS	TREATMENT
The fever causes nightmares accompanied by aggression, especially in children	Stramonium 15 CH 2 pillules 3 times a day
You are feverish, trembling, and exhausted, but not thirsty	Gelsemium 9 CH 2 pillules 3 times a day
The fever comes on with teething (particularly in babies) with one cheek red and hot and the other pale and cold, sometimes associated with greenish diarrhea	Chamomilla 9 CH 2 pillules 3 times a day
The fever comes on in bouts (high in the evening and not at all in the morning, or high for two days and not at all for one day, then, again, a high fever); you sweat and feel very tired	China rubra 5 CH (*Cinchona officinalis*) 2 pillules 3 times a day
You feel less feverish when you are still or in bed, and you are very thirsty	Bryonia 5 CH 2 pillules 3 times a day

INDICATIONS	TREATMENT
The fever is very high; you pass very little urine and are helped by cold compresses on the forehead; you feel bloated	Apis mellifica 5 CH 2 pillules 3 times a day
The fever is sudden and high, you are anxious even though still energetic, and you are not perspiring	Aconitum napellus 5 CH 2 pillules 3 times a day *to be stopped once the fever goes down*
The fever is high but your pulse remains slow	Pyrogenium 5 CH 2 pillules 3 times a day

ADVICE

Fever is a defense mechanism in the body when it is fighting an outside invader, most frequently viral or bacterial. Be careful, this is only a symptom: lowering the temperature may help, but is never enough to treat the problem. If the fever persists, a medical consultation is necessary in order to determine the cause. In the meantime, drink plenty of liquid, take cool baths to help lower your temperature, and do not cover yourself too much.

FISTULA, ANAL FISSURE

Elongated and superficial but very painful ulceration, located in the folds of the anus.

INDICATIONS	TREATMENT
The stools are acid and the fissures yellowish	Nitricum acidum 5 CH 2 pillules 3 times a day

INDICATIONS	TREATMENT
The whole digestive system suffers from acidity and burning	Iris versicolor 5 CH 2 pillules 3 times a day
There are small anal fissures	Argentum nitricum 5 CH 2 pillules 3 times a day
There are oozing hemorrhoids	Paeonia 5 CH 2 pillules 3 times a day
The stools contain mucus and are sometimes bloody	Mercurius corrosivus 5 CH 2 pillules 3 times a day
The anus is excessively red, burning, and painful	Belladonna 5 CH 2 pillules 3 times a day
The pain is better with heat (in a hot bath, for example)	Arsenicum album 5 CH 2 pillules 3 times a day

ADVICE

Avoid having an operation on an anal fissure. You risk relapse or secondary illnesses.

FLATULENCE, GAS

See: (eructations, burps), bloating, page 56.

FRACTURES

Sudden break of a bone. You fall or bump violently into something and you break a bone. It is very painful, and all movement becomes impossible.

INDICATIONS	TREATMENT
To treat the consequences of the trauma that caused the fracture	Arnica montana 9 CH 2 pillules 3 times a day
To reinforce the bones	Calcarea carbonicum 9 CH, Calcarea phosphorica 9 CH, Calcarea fluorica 9 CH 2 pillules 3 times a day *combined with* Silicea 9 CH 2 pillules 3 times a day
To accelerate healing of the bones	Symphytum 9 CH 2 pillules 3 times a day
For organotherapic treatment	Bones Total 4 CH 2 pillules 3 times a day

ADVICE

In case of fracture, an X-ray is indispensable, and immobilization often necessary. Surgery may be useful in case of serious displacement.

BOIL, CYST, PANARITIUM

See: Abscess, boil, panaritium, page 51.

GASTROENTERITIS

Acute, infectious inflammation of the stomach and intestines. You have stomach pain, you are vomiting, and you have diarrhea.

INDICATIONS	TREATMENT
The gastroenteritis is of viral origin, with nausea, diarrhea, and abdominal pains that are better with a hot water bottle placed on the stomach	Arsenicum album 5 CH 2 pillules 3 times a day
The gastroenteritis is due to food poisoning or a parasitic infestation; the person who is ill loses body awareness and cannot indicate precisely the source of the pain	Baptisia tinctoria 5 CH 2 pillules 3 times a day
All the preceding symptoms are accompanied by anxiety and agitation	Arsenicum album 15 CH 2 pillules 3 times a day
The vomiting is severe, ongoing, clear like water, and aggravated in the evening	Phosphorus 9 CH 1 dose every day for 3 days
The gastroenteritis appears after sudden dry cold	*Add to preceding remedies* Aconitum napellus 9 CH 2 pillules on going to bed
You sweat a great deal; you have a high temperature; you are tired	China rubra 5 CH (*Cinchona officinalis*) 2 pillules 3 times a day

INDICATIONS	TREATMENT
The gastroenteritis in a baby is due to lactose intolerance, not necessarily accompanied by diarrhea	Aethusa cynapium 5 CH 2 pillules 3 times a day *(to dissolve in the baby's bottle filled with water)*

See also: Diarrhea, page 135.

ADVICE

The main danger with gastroenteritis, especially in a child or an elderly person, is dehydration. Please make sure the sick persons drink plenty of liquids and adjust their diet as soon as they can eat again: preferably carrots, white rice, and bananas. You can also prepare a smoothie for children by mixing a banana with the water used to cook rice and a little sugar.

GAS

See: Flatulence (eructations, burps), bloating, page 56.

CHAPPED SKIN

Painful cracks in the skin, often located in the area of the lips or on the hands.

INDICATIONS	TREATMENT
LIPS	
The lips are chapped, you crave salt, and you are very thirsty	Natrum muriaticum 9 CH 1 dose a day for 3 days

INDICATIONS	TREATMENT
The corners of the lips are chapped, burning, and yellowish	Natrum muriaticum 9 CH 1 dose a day for 3 days *combined with* Nitricum acidum 5 CH 2 pillules 3 times a day
You are very thirsty (for large quantities of water); you are constipated; your skin is dry	Bryonia 5 CH 2 pillules 3 times a day
HANDS	
Your skin is dry and delicate	Alumina 5 CH 2 pillules 3 times a day
The chapping appears in winter	Petroleum 5 CH 2 pillules 3 times a day
Your skin peels and you feel better with warm compresses	Arsenicum album 5 CH 2 pillules 3 times a day
The chapping turns into fissures, with a honey-like secretion followed by crusts	Graphites 5 CH 2 pillules 3 times a day
You have alcoholic tendencies	Sulphuricum acidum 5 CH 2 pillules 3 times a day

ADVICE

To prevent chapped lips, make sure that they are not continuously wet. Avoid pacifiers for children, and dry your lips regularly if you tend to have a lot of saliva.

GINGIVITIS

Inflammation of the gums. They are red and bleed easily. You have a lot of saliva, you may have bad breath, and the least contact with food causes pain.

INDICATIONS	TREATMENT
The gums are very red, inflamed, and painful	Belladonna 5 CH 2 pillules 3 times a day
Your tongue is white and retains the imprint of the teeth, you have a lot of saliva and bad breath	Mercurius solubilis 5 CH 2 pillules 3 times a day
There are small ulcerations in the gums	Mercurius corrosivus 5 CH 2 pillules 3 times a day
The ulcerations are deep and are aggravated by sugary foods	Argentum nitricum 5 CH 2 pillules 3 times a day *combined with* Kalium bichromicum 5 CH 2 pillules 3 times a day
You bleed a lot	Phosphorus 9 CH 2 pillules 3 times a day

ADVICE

In all cases, to improve oral hygiene, you can use Calendula and Phytolacca mother tinctures as a mouthwash, 20 drops of each in a small amount of water.

SWELLING OF FINGERS

The ring mark, when the fingers swell so much that they prevent you from taking off a ring that you put on with no problem that same morning or the day before.

INDICATIONS	TREATMENT
You have rheumatic pain; you do not tolerate humidity well	Natrum sulphuricum 5 CH 2 pillules 3 times a day
Your fingers are very swollen and painful	Bovista 5 CH 2 pillules 3 times a day
Your fingers swell due to an allergy or an insect bite or sting	Apis mellifica 9 CH 2 pillules 3 times a day

ADVICE

To remove rings that fit too tightly around swollen fingers, here's a simple home remedy: soap your hands well under very cold water until you can gently slide the rings off.

GOUT

Acute inflammation of the joints, skin, or kidneys, due to excess uric acid. This condition is often hereditary.

INDICATIONS	TREATMENT
In all cases	Drainage remedy for liver and kidneys *(See: Complex remedies, page 320)* 10 drops 3 times a day *combined with* Erigeron canadensis mother tincture 10 drops 3 times a day *and* Lycopodium 5 CH 2 pillules 3 times a day *and* Uricum acidum 5 CH 2 pillules 3 times a day *and* Colchicum 5 CH 2 pillules 3 times a day
Your small joints are inflamed; your urine output has diminished	Benzoicum acidum 5 CH 2 pillules 3 times a day
Your small joints are inflamed by the calcium deposits	Calcarea carbonica 5 CH 2 pillules 3 times a day
Your pain is better with cold or the applications of ice	Ledum palustre 5 CH 2 pillules 3 times a day

ADVICE

Gout is mainly an ailment of men who are healthy, like to eat well, and have a tendency toward excess in food and drink. One would advise, of course, a review of their diet, giving preference to lighter and healthier foods and limiting fatty foods, offal, and alcohol, particularly white wine. Drink a lot of spring water.

FLU

Viral illness, infectious and contagious, which can spread into an epidemic. You have a combination of fever, muscle pain, headaches, and tiredness. All these can be accompanied by rhinitis or bronchitis.

INDICATIONS	TREATMENT
TO PREVENT THE FLU	
In all cases	Influenzinum 9 CH 1 dose a week in October *then* 5 to 8 pillules a month until February
To stimulate immune defenses	*Add* Serum Yersin 9 CH 1 dose a week in October *then* 1 dose a month until February *combined with* Thymuline 9 CH 1 dose a week in October *then* 1 dose a month until February
TO TREAT THE FLU	
In all cases	Influenzinum 9 CH 1 dose a day for 3 days *then* Influenzinum (strain for that year) 15 CH 1 dose on the 4th day
The flu appears after sudden, dry cold, and you do not perspire	*Add* Aconitum napellus 9 CH 2 pillules 3 times a day

INDICATIONS	TREATMENT
You sweat and your temperature remains between 100°F and 102°F	*Add* Belladonna 9 CH 2 pillules 3 times a day
You are starting to become delirious, especially at night	*Add* Belladonna 15 CH 2 pillules 3 times a day
You just have the flu with muscle pain; you find your bed too hard	*Add* Arnica montana 9 CH 2 pillules 3 times a day
The pain is more extreme; your bones are painful; your eyes are sensitive to touch	*Add* Eupatorium perfoliatum 5 CH 2 pillules 3 times a day
You are exhausted by a high fever and you tremble; you are not thirsty	*Add* Gelsemium 5 CH 2 pillules 3 times a day
You feel good lying in bed; it is no use waking you; you like to rest; you feel less bad lying on the painful side; you are thirsty for large quantities of water	*Add* Bryonia 5 CH 2 pillules 3 times a day
Your temperature is fluctuating; you perspire a lot and are tired, with, possibly, diarrhea and nausea	*Add* China rubra 5 CH (*Cinchona officinalis*) 2 pillules 3 times a day
You feel better when you are moving about	*Add* Rhus toxicodendron 5 CH 2 pillules 3 times a day

INDICATIONS	TREATMENT
TO RECOVER FROM THE FLU	
To regain appetite in case of intense tiredness	China rubra 5 CH (*Cinchona officinalis*) 2 pillules 3 times a day
To convalesce more quickly	Rosa canina macerate of the bud (glycerinated) 20 drops 3 times a day *combined with* Ribes nigrum macerate of the bud (glycerinated) 30 drops 3 times a day *and* Ginseng mother tincture 20 drops 3 times a day
You have lost weight in spite of having a good appetite	Natrum muriaticum 5 CH 2 pillules 3 times a day
You remain chilly; your hands and feet are always cold	Silicea 5 CH 2 pillules 3 times a day

INDICATIONS	TREATMENT
For a child or an adolescent who has grown a great deal during the flu and is very tired after it	Kalium phosphoricum 5 CH 2 pillules 3 times a day

ADVICE

The flu vaccine, widely publicized every autumn, is very strong and entails all the inconveniences of a standard vaccine. It would be better to limit it to people who are weak (the elderly, diabetics, cardiac patients). For others, reinforcing the immune system at the beginning of winter is often quite adequate to get you through it.

PREGNANCY

Everything that happens in the mother's body between the time of conception and giving birth. You are going to have a baby. Your body is transformed and undergoes considerable physical and hormonal changes, not always without some minor inconveniences.

INDICATIONS	TREATMENT
IN ALL CASES	
To help you stay healthy during pregnancy	Schuessler Tissue Salts 6 DH 3 tablets 3 times a day

INDICATIONS	TREATMENT
CONSTIPATION	
You are constipated	Bryonia 5 CH 2 pillules 3 times a day *combined with* Alumina 5 CH 2 pillules 3 times a day
CIRCULATION	
You have hemorrhoids	Aesculus hippocastanum 5 CH 2 pillules 3 times a day *combined with* Hamamelis 5 CH 2 pillules 3 times a day
You have hemorrhoids and weakening of the sphincter	Aloe 5 CH 2 pillules 3 times a day
You have hemorrhoids and heavy legs	Collinsonia canadensis 9 CH 2 pillules 3 times a day
You have varicose veins	Calcarea fluorica 5 CH 2 pillules 3 times a day
NAUSEA	
You are nauseated and do not feel better after vomiting	Ipecac 5 CH 2 pillules 3 times a day
You are nauseated and your food preferences change (you can no longer bear coffee, which you used to love; you crave oysters, which you used to detest)	Ipecac 5 CH 2 pillules 3 times a day *combined with* Ignatia amara 5 CH 2 pillules 3 times a day

INDICATIONS	TREATMENT
The smell of tobacco turns your stomach and gives you vertigo	Tabacum 5 CH 2 pillules 3 times a day
Nausea accompanied by cough	Lobelia inflata 5 CH 2 pillules 3 times a day
You are anxious and agitated; you suffer from diarrhea and nausea	Arsenicum album 9 CH 2 pillules 3 times a day
ACIDITY	
You have acid reflux	Robinia 5 CH 2 pillules 3 times a day
You feel acidity in the whole digestive tract, from the esophagus to the anus	Iris versicolor 5 CH 2 pillules 3 times a day
You have acid reflux, especially between 4 and 8 p.m., and liver problems	Lycopodium 5 CH 2 pillules 3 times a day
WATER RETENTION	
You have water retention all over your body	Natrum sulphuricum 5 CH 2 pillules 3 times a day *combined with* Orthosiphon mother tincture 20 drops 3 times a day
You have water retention only in the lower body, and you have cellulite	Thuja occidentalis 5 CH 2 pillules 3 times a day *combined with* Orthosiphon mother tincture 20 drops 3 times a day

INDICATIONS	TREATMENT
You have water retention only in the fingers, the lips, or the face	Bovista 5 CH 2 pillules 3 times a day *combined with* Orthosiphon mother tincture 20 drops 3 times a day
NERVOUSNESS	
You are anxious and very agitated between 1 and 3 a.m.	Arsenicum album 9 CH 2 pillules 3 times a day
You are depressed, you are tense, and you have a chloasma	Sepia 9 CH 2 pillules 3 times a day *or* Natrum muriaticum 9 CH 2 pillules 3 times a day
You are tense and in a gloomy mood and have a urinary tract infection	Sepia 9 CH 2 pillules 3 times a day *combined with* Colibacillinum 5 CH (*Bacillus coli*) 2 pillules 3 times a day *alternating with* Serum anticolibacillaire 5 CH 2 pillules 3 times a day *and with* Formica rufa 5 CH 2 pillules 3 times a day
You are tense, in a gloomy mood, and you have serious cystitis	*Add* Cantharis 5 CH 2 pillules 3 times a day

INDICATIONS	TREATMENT
BEFORE THE BIRTH	
To avoid anxiety before and during the birth	Gelsemium 9 CH 1 dose at the start of labor 1 dose during the birth
You are strong and of carbonic constitution	*A few days before the birth* Calcarea carbonica 5 CH 2 pillules 3 times a day
To accelerate the dilation of the cervix	*From the start of labor* Caulophyllum 5 CH 2 pillules every 10 minutes *combined with* Actaea racemosa 5 CH 2 pillules every hour
In case of an epidural	Hypericum perforatum 5 CH 1 dose before the birth
In case of a cesarean or an episiotomy	Staphysagria 5 CH 1 dose once the cesarean is decided upon
If you are given an anesthetic	Nux vomica 5 CH 1 dose as soon as possible
AFTER THE BIRTH	
In all cases	Arnica montana 9 CH 2 pillules 3 times a day
You have been anesthetized; you are worn out during the day; you are very agitated at night; you are constipated	Opium 9 CH 2 pillules 3 times a day

INDICATIONS	TREATMENT
You have undergone a cesarean or an episiotomy	Staphysagria 5 CH 2 pillules 3 times a day
POSTPARTUM DEPRESSION	
You feel depressed after the birth	Arnica montana 9 CH 2 pillules 3 times a day *combined with* Sepia 9 CH 2 pillules 3 times a day
You close in on yourself; you cannot express your discomfort and have the impression of being forsaken	Staphysagria 9 CH 2 pillules 3 times a day
You tremble; you are anxious	Gelsemium 9 CH 2 pillules 3 times a day
You burst into tears	Ambra grisea 9 CH 2 pillules 3 times a day

See also: Flatulence (eructations, burps), bloating, page 56; Cramps, page 125; Pain—back, page 143.

ADVICE

I do not know any allopathic medicine that is not toxic to the pregnant woman or her baby. Even antiemetics given as a matter of course can be a source of problems, including if they appear harmless to the fetus. They tend to induce somnolence and trembling in the mother. It is even more ludicrous to prescribe neuroleptics or antidepressants to the mother subject to excitation or depression. Pregnancy is a perfect example of when you should only use homeopathic remedies, as far as possible.

HANGOVER

Consequences of too much alcohol. You have drunk one, two, or three glasses too many. You have a headache, furry tongue, and bad breath. You are sleepy or light-headed.

INDICATIONS	TREATMENT
To prevent or treat a hangover	Nux vomica 5 CH 2 pillules before the party 2 pillules after the party
You have a good meal when you drink alcohol: to avoid indigestion	Antimonium crudum 5 CH 2 pillules before the meal 2 pillules after the meal

ADVICE

To help you to recover, drink a lot of water and eat bread and fruits: their slow sugars will do you good. Also consider the very dangerous consequences of excessive consumption of alcohol. Completely avoid driving. Do not make a habit of drinking too much: you can become an alcoholic without realizing it.

HEMATOMA

See: Bruise, hematoma, page 89.

HEMORRHOIDS

See: Circulation (problems with) varicose veins, heavy legs, hemorrhoids, page 108.

HEPATITIS (VIRAL OR TOXIC)

With inflammation of the liver, of viral and infectious or toxic origin, after the absorption of medicines, for example. Your skin has a yellow tinge.

INDICATIONS	TREATMENT
In all cases	Phosphorus 9 CH 1 dose a week for 1 month *or* 2 pillules 3 times a day for 1 month *then* Phosphorus 12 CH 1 dose a week for 1 month *or* 2 pillules 3 times a day for 1 month *then* Phosphorus 15 CH 1 dose a week for 1 month *or* 2 pillules twice a day for 1 month
To detoxify the liver	Nux vomica 5 CH 2 pillules 3 times a day *combined with* General drainage remedy for the liver *(See: Complex remedies, page 320)* 20 drops 3 times a day
The hepatitis is chronic; there is an aggravation of symptoms between 4 and 8 p.m.	Lycopodium 9 CH 2 pillules 3 times a day

INDICATIONS	TREATMENT
The hepatitis is due to taking medicine	*Combine with the preceding remedy* Isotherapic of the medicine concerned 5 CH *if the hepatitis is recent; in the highest potency if it is long-standing* 2 pillules 3 times a day

ADVICE

Before treating hepatitis, it is essential to make a full examination (ultrasound of liver, scan, bioassay, and so on) to understand its origin. Simple acetaminophen may be the cause of hepatitis. I have achieved cures with the isotherapic of acetaminophen combined with Phosphorus, Nux vomica, and Opium, with patients already in a pre-comatose state.

HERPES

Viral attack causing skin problems characterized by the appearance of one or many vesicles (in clusters). It burns, pricks, and itches; rarely looks attractive; and is always contagious.

INDICATIONS	TREATMENT
IN CASE OF AN OUTBREAK	
Whether it is skin or vaginal herpes	Vaccinotoxinum 9 CH 1 dose a day for 3 days *combined with* Rhus toxicodendron 5 CH 2 pillules 3 times a day
Genital herpes accompanied by itching	Croton tiglium 5 CH 2 pillules 3 times a day

INDICATIONS	TREATMENT
The vesicles ooze a syrupy liquid	Vaccinotoxinum 9 CH 1 dose a day for 3 days *combined with* Mezereum 5 CH 2 pillules 3 times a day
There is inflammation with edema	Apis mellifica 5 CH 2 pillules 3 times a day
You have intense burning sensations, aggravated at night; better with applied heat—a hot water bottle or a compress	Arsenicum album 5 CH 2 pillules 3 times a day
The herpes is painful, with large, burning blisters	Cantharis 5 CH 2 pillules 3 times a day
Dry herpes, aggravated by the ocean	Natrum muriaticum 5 CH 2 pillules 3 times a day
Your skin is not healthy; you often feel too hot; water and heat increase the itching	Sulfur 5 CH 2 pillules 3 times a day
IN CASE OF LABIAL HERPES (COLD SORE)	
The sore has some pus, a syrupy, yellowish substance	Staphylococcinum 9 CH 2 pillules 3 times a day *or* Pyrogenium 5 CH 2 pillules 3 times a day

INDICATIONS	TREATMENT
The blister oozes	*To accelerate the secretion* Hepar sulphur 5 CH 2 pillules 3 times a day *or to regulate the secretion* Hepar sulphur 9 CH 2 pillules 3 times a day *in combination with* Pyrogenium 9 CH 2 pillules 3 times a day
The cold sores are accompanied by small cracks around the lips	Nitricum acidum 5 CH 2 pillules 3 times a day
FOR DEEP-ACTING TREATMENT	
The herpes appears systematically in the presence of something that triggers it: ocean, mountains, sun	Vaccinotoxinum 9 CH 1 dose every month *and* 1 dose a day for 2 days before departure
The herpes appears routinely in the sun	*Add* Apis mellifica 5 CH 2 pillules 3 times a day
The herpes appears routinely by the sea	*Add* Natrum muriaticum 5 CH 2 pillules 3 times a day
The herpes appears routinely before your period	*Add* Folliculinum 9 CH 1 dose on the 14th and 21st days of cycle

ADVICE

Deep-acting treatment is essential because this is an illness you do not recover from. The virus responsible, harbored in the lymph nodes, produces flare-ups at shorter or longer intervals, and these may or may not be caused by different situations (stress, tiredness, periods). Protect yourself and protect those close to you in case of a crisis: herpes is very contagious (avoid embracing or touching those close to you). Genital herpes is even classed as a sexually transmitted disease (it is essential to use a condom for any sexual contact during flare-ups).

HICCUPS

Spasmodic contraction of the diaphragm, causing an abrupt inhalation accompanied by a characteristic noise on the closure of the glottis.

INDICATIONS	TREATMENT
To treat the spasm during the attack	Cuprum metallicum 5 CH 2 pillules every 10 minutes
To treat the spasm, with deep-acting treatment	Cuprum metallicum 5 CH 2 pillules 3 times a day *alternate with* Magnesia phosphorica 5 CH 2 pillules 3 times a day *or* Nux vomica 5 CH 2 pillules 3 times a day

ADVICE

To end the attack, you can also try one or two home remedies: hold your breath for as long as possible (to restore the rhythm of the diaphragm), drink a glass of cold water very slowly and without breathing (works quite well), or make yourself undergo a shock, whether thermal (an ice cube down your back) or emotional (by asking an acquaintance to frighten you). But it has to be said that results of the latter method are fairly random.

HYPERACTIVITY

See: Excitation, hyperactivity, page 159.

MENTAL AND EMOTIONAL HYPERSENSITIVITY

Exaggerated reactions when confronted with certain situations.

INDICATIONS	TREATMENT
All your senses are hypersensitive: you cannot tolerate even a sheet covering you, light, odors, or noise	Nux vomica 9 CH 2 pillules 3 times a day
You cannot bear any light, but, paradoxically, you feel worse at night, from the time you go to bed	Hyoscyamus niger 9 CH 2 pillules 3 times a day
You are hypersensitive to strong light	Belladonna 9 CH 2 pillules 3 times a day
You cannot bear strong light (to the point of it making you furious), but you are calmed by soft light	Stramonium 9 CH 2 pillules 3 times a day

INDICATIONS	TREATMENT
You are hypersensitive to sounds; you cannot bear any noise, especially the tick-tock of a clock or the drip-drip of a leaky faucet	Theridion 9 CH 2 pillules 3 times a day
You are hypersensitive to movement, noise, odors, light, and also to annoyances	Ignatia amara 9 CH 2 pillules 3 times a day
Your hypersensitivity causes suppressed anger; you cannot express what you feel	Staphysagria 9 CH 2 pillules 3 times a day
Your hypersensitivity induces spasms in the abdomen, with colitis and inflammation	Colocynthis 9 CH 2 pillules 3 times a day
You are hypersensitive to estrogen (you become very irritable before your period, and everything improves when it starts)	Folliculinum 9 CH 2 pillules 3 times a day

See also: Emotionalism, hypersensitivity, page 151.

ADVICE

Go over situations that cause you difficulty and try to train yourself to control your emotions in these particular cases. Certain behavioral psychology techniques could help.

HYPERTENSION

High blood pressure, leading to cardiac and circulatory pathologies.

INDICATIONS	TREATMENT
Your hypertension comes on in bouts; your skin becomes red	Orthosiphon mother tincture (diuretic rich in potassium) 50 drops 3 times a day *combined with* Belladonna 5 CH 2 pillules 3 times a day
Your hypertension comes on in bouts; you have a pulsating feeling in your temples	Glonoine 5 CH 2 pillules 3 times a day
You have profuse urine	Lespedeza mother tincture 50 drops 3 times a day
You have a high content of uric acid	Erigeron canadensis mother tincture 50 drops 3 times a day
You are overweight and are on a diet	Pilosella mother tincture 50 drops 3 times a day
You suffer from demineralization	Horsetail (*Equisetum arvense*), a diuretic rich in Silica, mother tincture 50 drops 3 times a day
You are nervous, stressed, and intensely intellectual, but you do no physical exercise	Nux vomica 9 CH 2 pillules 3 times a day
You are hyperactive and agitated	Argentum nitricum 9 CH 2 pillules 3 times a day

INDICATIONS	TREATMENT
You are a food and wine enthusiast (like to eat and drink well)	Hepatorenal Drainage remedy *(See: Complex remedies, page 320)* 50 drops 3 times a day *combined with* Sulfur 9 CH 2 pillules 3 times a day
Your hypertension is accompanied by anemia and often constipation	Plumbum 5 CH 2 pillules 3 times a day
You have water retention in your whole body	Natrum sulphuricum 9 CH 2 pillules 3 times a day
You have water retention localized in one part of your body	Apis mellifica 9 CH 2 pillules 3 times a day
The water retention is concentrated in the lower limbs	Thuja occidentalis 5 CH 2 pillules 3 times a day
You have water retention because of cortisone	*Add to preceding remedies* Cortisone 9 CH 1 dose a week *combined with* Ribes nigrum, glycerinated tincture of macerated bud 50 drops 3 times a day

ADVICE

It is essential to see a doctor. Preferably consult a homeopathic cardiologist. This illness is often brought on by being overweight, a sedentary lifestyle, or stress. Be careful to eat healthy food, do some physical activity, and avoid stressful situations as much as possible. And stop smoking!

NEONATAL JAUNDICE (YELLOW SKIN IN A NEWBORN)

Yellowish color of the baby's skin, due to an accumulation of bilirubin.

INDICATIONS	TREATMENT
In all cases	Phosphorus 9 CH 2 pillules 3 times a day *(to dissolve in the baby's bottle)*

ADVICE

No need to panic: jaundice is common in babies in the days after birth and absolutely normal. If you are breastfeeding your child, you can take the remedy yourself. It will pass the blood barrier and thereby treat the child.

IMPOTENCE

Physical inability in a man to perform the sexual act, due to lack of erection.

INDICATIONS	TREATMENT
AT THE TIME	
To avoid failure	Badiaga 9 CH 2 pillules 3 times a day
To facilitate the dilatation of the penis and the erection	Yohimbinum mother tincture 20 drops 3 times a day

INDICATIONS	TREATMENT
The impotence follows tiredness after an illness or traumatic event	Selenium 9 CH 2 pillules 3 times a day *combined with* Arnica montana 9 CH 2 pillules 3 times a day
The impotence is accompanied by a loss of memory and general weakness	Phosphoricum acidum 9 CH 2 pillules 3 times a day
The impotence is due to mental tiredness and excessive masturbation	Kalium phosphoricum 9 CH 2 pillules 3 times a day
The impotence is due to overwork and a diet that is too rich	Nux vomica 9 CH 2 pillules 3 times a day
FOR DEEP-ACTING TREATMENT	
At mealtimes, your eyes are bigger than your stomach, your abdomen is bloated (flatulence), and you would very much like to continue eating, but you cannot; you never satisfy your partners (soft erections) in spite of desire	Lycopodium 9 CH 2 pillules 3 times a day

See also: Premature ejaculation, page 149.

ADVICE

There are not only psychological factors involved in erectile dysfunction; physical aspects may also contribute, like insufficiency of blood flow in the penis. A consultation with a specialist will help you address your particular issues.

FECAL INCONTINENCE

Impossible to retain stools. You don't even have time to get to the toilet.

INDICATIONS	TREATMENT
IN CHILDREN	
Fecal incontinence appears after a traumatic event, mental/emotional or physical	Arnica montana 9 CH 2 pillules 3 times a day
Fecal incontinence appears because the child cannot express discomfort	Staphysagria 9 CH 2 pillules 3 times a day
IN ADULTS	
Fecal incontinence is due to weakened sphincters, causing leaks during flatulence or with the slightest motion of the sphincter muscles	Aloe 5 CH 2 pillules 3 times a day
Fecal incontinence is due to weakness of sphincters, causing leaks when you cough or laugh	Causticum 5 CH 2 pillules 3 times a day
Fecal incontinence is connected to a sense of abandonment, especially in elderly people or young children	Staphysagria 9 CH 2 pillules 3 times a day

You should adopt a diet that hardens your stools a bit to limit the problem. Eat a lot of white rice and bananas, and quince jelly at breakfast.

INDIGESTION AFTER EXCESSIVE EATING

Sudden but transitory dysfunction of the digestive system. You have eaten too much or too well, you have abdominal pain, you are nauseated, and you have headaches.

INDICATIONS	TREATMENT
To drain the liver and eliminate the excess	Complex remedy containing at least three of the following remedies in low dilution: Chelidonium majus, Taxaracum, Carduus marianus, Boldo, Solidago, Berberis vulgaris, Chrysanthemum americanum *(See: Complex remedies, page 320)* 2 pillules 3 times a day
You have a tendency to eat too much; you have stomach pain, heaviness, a white tongue, and maybe nausea	Antimonium crudum 5 CH 2 pillules at the time of the indigestion *combined with* Calcarea carbonicum 9 CH 1 dose a week
You have also drunk too much and crash after a meal	Nux vomica 5 CH 2 pillules at the time of the indigestion

ADVICE

Being moderate in all things, at mealtime as elsewhere, will guard you against many misadventures.

STAPHYLOCOCCUS INFECTION

Pathogenic development of *Staphylococcus* in the system.

INDICATIONS	TREATMENT
Staphylococcus causes skin problems (acne, boils, abscess)	Lappa major mother tincture 10 drops 3 times a day *combined with* Staphylococcinum 9 CH 2 pillules 3 times a day *and* Pyrogenium 9 CH 2 pillules 3 times a day
When the infection is almost over	Sulfur 9 CH 1 dose

ADVICE

If the infection is due to *Staphylococcus aureus*, antibiotics are necessary (in addition to homeopathic treatment).

URINARY TRACT INFECTION

See: Cystitis, urinary tract infection, page 127.

TONSILLITIS

See: Sore throat, tonsillitis, throat pain, pharyngitis, page 67.

SUNSTROKE

You have been exposed to the sun for too long; you suffer from sunstroke and sunburn, headaches, vertigo, nausea.

INDICATIONS	TREATMENT
You are hot and have a red face and dilatation of the pupils; you cannot tolerate light; you have a fever; you are sweating; you are thirsty	Belladonna 9 CH 2 pillules 3 times a day
In addition to the preceding symptoms, you are delirious	Belladonna 15 CH 2 pillules 3 times a day
You have pulsating temples	Glonoine 5 CH 2 pillules 3 times a day
You are worn out and feel stupid; you have a high temperature and are exhausted by sunstroke; you tremble; you are not thirsty	Gelsemium 9 CH 2 pillules 3 times a day
Sunstroke makes you debilitated	Natrum carbonicum 5 CH 2 pillules 3 times a day
You have a high fever but do not perspire; you feel anxious and agitated	Aconitum napellus 9 CH 2 pillules 3 times a day

ADVICE

It is crucial to rehydrate yourself in case of sunstroke, even if you are not thirsty. Drink plenty of cool water, try to stay in a cool place, and take a cool shower or bath.

FOOD POISONING

Dysfunction of the digestive system. You have eaten food that was indigestible because it was spoiled or it contained bacteria (mayonnaise that has been out of the refrigerator for too long, a bad oyster, and so on). You have pain in the head and the stomach; you vomit and are feverish.

INDICATIONS	TREATMENT
You are tired; you have nausea and diarrhea	China rubra 5 CH (*Cinchona officinalis*) 2 pillules 3 times a day
You feel uneasy when you get diarrhea; you sweat a great deal and have vertigo	Veratrum album 5 CH 2 pillules 3 times a day
You are overcome by delirium, particularly after salmonella poisoning	Paratyphoidinum B 9 CH 2 pillules 3 times a day
You suffer from mental confusion	Baptisia tinctoria 9 CH 2 pillules 3 times a day
In all cases	*Add* Liver Drainage *(See: Complex remedies, page 320)* 20 drops 3 times a day

ADVICE

Avoid dehydration in the case of nausea and serious diarrhea accompanied by perspiration. If possible, drink a lot of liquids—alternating sweet and savory drinks, regularly: tea with honey, then vegetable bouillon, fruit juice, tomato juice with celery salt, and so on.

DRUNKENNESS

Abuse of alcohol, altered perception and behavior. Your sight becomes blurred, you lose your balance, your head spins, and your mood is changeable (you can become violent, euphoric, or very sad all of a sudden). You lose control of yourself and your reactions.

INDICATIONS	TREATMENT
A single episode of alcohol abuse resulting in sleepiness	Nux vomica 5 CH 2 pillules 3 times a day
Drunkenness is chronic, social, from boredom or resentment	Lachesis 9 CH 2 pillules 3 times a day
For people who are addicted to alcohol who can drink anything and everything	Capsicum 5 CH 2 pillules 3 times a day *combined with* Sulphuricum Acidum 5 CH 2 pillules 3 times a day
To support the liver of an alcoholic	Sulphuricum Acidum 5 CH 2 pillules 3 times a day
The alcoholic is puffy, red, and blotchy; their liver is affected	Phosphorus 9 CH 2 pillules 3 times a day
The alcoholic is violent	Stramonium 5 CH 2 pillules 3 times a day
As a deep-acting remedy	Syphilinum 9 CH 2 pillules 3 times a day
As a remedy for a crisis	Ethylicum 5 CH 2 pillules 3 times a day

ADVICE

If it remains an occasional problem, drunkenness brings only a minor risk of real threats to health. Nevertheless, it may degenerate into serious situations (accidents, aggressiveness, and so on), so it is preferable to limit the occasions when you get drunk, and if it does happen, counteract the drunkenness and reduce the effects as soon as possible or stay in bed!

JEALOUSY

Feelings of resentment or desire that a person feels toward others who have what they would like to have for themselves.

INDICATIONS	TREATMENT
You are morbidly jealous; you talk a lot about all sorts of subjects concerning your jealousy; you drink a little	Lachesis 9 CH 2 pillules 3 times a day
You suffer from suppressed jealousy and do not express yourself	Natrum muriaticum 9 CH 2 pillules 3 times a day *or* 1 dose a week
You suffer from suppressed jealousy; you do not express yourself; it manifests pathologically (eruption of acne, anorexia, ulcers)	Staphysagria 9 CH 1 dose a week

INDICATIONS	TREATMENT
The jealousy makes you verbally aggressive; you feel like screaming	Nux vomica 9 CH 2 pillules 3 times a day
The jealousy makes you physically aggressive	Mercurius solubilis 9 CH 2 pillules 3 times a day
The jealousy makes you verbally and physically aggressive	Stramonium 9 CH 2 pillules 3 times a day

ADVICE

Learn to trust in yourself at first and then in other people as well.

HEAVY LEGS

See: Circulation (problems with), page 108.

CYSTS

See: Abscess, boil, panaritium, page 51.

OVARIAN CYST

Small sac in the shape of a ball, located on the ovary.

INDICATIONS	TREATMENT
The cyst is located on the right ovary	Lycopodium 5 CH 2 pillules 3 times a day *or* Palladium 5 CH 2 pillules 3 times a day

INDICATIONS	TREATMENT
The cyst is located on the left ovary	Lachesis 5 CH 2 pillules 3 times a day or Thuja occidentalis 5 CH 2 pillules 3 times a day
In all cases, to ensure hormonal regulation	Ovarinum 4 CH 2 pillules 3 times a day

ADVICE

In all cases, a precise diagnosis is essential to avoid missing diagnosis of a serious illness. Allopathic treatment may prove necessary along with homeopathy.

LARYNGITIS

Acute or chronic inflammation of the larynx. Your throat feels rough, and this very irritating condition causes a hoarse cough.

INDICATIONS	TREATMENT
Your throat feels rough; you feel pain as if there were a needle in it, sometimes with small ulcerations	Argentum nitricum 5 CH 2 pillules 3 times a day *or if you are very agitated* Argentum nitricum 9 CH 2 pillules 3 times a day
You suffer from laryngitis after having talked for too long	Arnica montana 9 CH 2 pillules 3 times a day

INDICATIONS	TREATMENT
Your laryngitis is painful and accompanied by hoarseness: it causes your voice to change from high to low; it breaks on one note or high intonation and you are unable to control it	Arum triphyllum 5 CH 2 pillules 3 times a day
Your voice improves from speaking a little	Rhus toxicodendron 5 CH 2 pillules 3 times a day
Your voice is better by the ocean	Bromum 5 CH 2 pillules 3 times a day
Your throat is irritated and scratchy, which causes a cough	Rumex crispus 5 CH 2 pillules 3 times a day
Your cough is spasmodic, an asthma-like cough	Badiaga 5 CH 2 pillules 3 times a day
Your cough is wheezy and hollow; you have difficulty breathing, especially at night before midnight	Spongia tosta 5 CH 2 pillules 3 times a day
You are hoarse, especially in the morning, with a hoarse cough and burning sensations; it is better with drinking	Causticum 5 CH 2 pillules 3 times a day

INDICATIONS	TREATMENT
For a child with a blocked nose who coughs and has difficulty breathing, especially at night	Sambucus nigra 5 CH 2 pillules 3 times a day
If you smoke	Tabacum 5 CH 2 pillules 3 times a day *combined with* Lobelia inflata 5 CH 2 pillules 3 times a day

See also: Hoarseness, aphonia, page 153.

ADVICE

Keep your throat warm and eat honey to temporarily calm the irritation.

DRY, CHAPPED LIPS

Cracking of the lips, occurring mainly when the lips are dry

INDICATIONS	TREATMENT
Your lips are naturally dry and cracked	Natrum muriaticum 5 CH 2 pillules 3 times a day
The chapping is worse in winter, with a vertical fissure on the lower lip, which can bleed	Natrum muriaticum 5 CH 2 pillules 3 times a day
The chapping looks blackish and is worse in winter; you have digestive problems or nausea	Petroleum 5 CH 2 pillules 3 times a day

INDICATIONS	TREATMENT
There are yellowish fissures at the corners of the lips	Nitricum acidum 5 CH 2 pillules 3 times a day
Your lips are chapped because you are blowing your nose a lot	Arum triphyllum 5 CH 2 pillules 3 times a day
Your lips are also slightly swollen and you are not thirsty	Apis mellifica 5 CH 2 pillules 3 times a day
Your lips are chapped because of acid reflux	Iris versicolor 5 CH 2 pillules 3 times a day *combined with* Muriaticum acidum 5 CH 2 pillules 3 times a day

ADVICE

A greasy balm applied regularly soothes the discomfort of chapped lips.

LOGORRHEA

Tendency to talk continuously.

INDICATIONS	TREATMENT
You speak continuously, following your train of thought	Lachesis 9 CH 2 pillules 3 times a day
You talk a lot, going off in all directions	Actaea racemosa 9 CH 2 pillules 3 times a day

Shhhh! For once, listen to me! Logorrhea can be a real pathology and a source of embarrassment for your family and friends. What are you hiding behind this flood of words? What if you spoke about it to a psychologist?

LOW BACK PAIN

Lower back pain coming on suddenly.

INDICATIONS	TREATMENT
The pain is due to a wrong move	Arnica montana 9 CH 2 pillules 3 times a day
You are in pain from the slightest movement, and you support yourself in bed on the painful side	Bryonia 5 CH 2 pillules 3 times a day
You feel better when you move	Rhus toxicodendron 5 CH 2 pillules 3 times a day
You have an asymmetric constitution	*Add to preceding remedies* Calcarea fluorica 5 CH 2 pillules 3 times a day
In all cases, to counteract the inflammation	Harpagophytum (Devil's Claw) mother tincture 20 drops 3 times a day

ADVICE

Spare your back!

- Avoid mattresses that are too soft.

- Do not bend over to pick something up; bend your knees.

- ✎ When you are working at a computer or at the office, do not bend forward.

- ✎ Always warm up before exercise.

- ✎ Walk or swim, but avoid tennis, skiing, and parachuting.

DISLOCATION

Displacement of a joint, often after a blow or a wrong move

INDICATIONS	TREATMENT
The dislocation is due to a blow or a traumatic event	Arnica montana 9 CH 2 pillules 3 times a day
The tendons are affected	Ruta graveolens 5 CH 2 pillules 3 times a day
You feel better with complete rest	Bryonia 5 CH 2 pillules 3 times a day
You suffer from repeated dislocations	Syphilinum 9 CH 1 dose a month *combined with* Calcarea fluorica 9 CH 1 dose a week

ADVICE

Start by seeing a physiotherapist or an osteopath, who will put things back in place.

CLAMMY HANDS

Continual perspiration of the hands, permanently clammy.

INDICATIONS	TREATMENT
You sweat a lot because you are agitated and you are trying too hard; you like the high life and living it up	Sulfur 9 CH 2 pillules 3 times a day
You also have a lot of saliva, especially at night, and you can tolerate neither heat nor cold	Mercurius solubilis 7 CH 2 pillules 3 times a day
Your hands and feet are clammy, but you are chilly	Silicea 5 CH 2 pillules 3 times a day
Your whole body is sweaty	Pilocarpus jaborandi 5 CH 2 pillules 3 times a day
You also have cellulite	Thuja occidentalis 5 CH 2 pillules 3 times a day

ADVICE

Keep a little talcum powder nearby and rub your palms with it regularly. That will at least allow you to greet your colleagues without feeling embarrassed.

BACK PAIN

See: Low back pain, page 211.

HEADACHE

Pain radiating all over the head or in one part of the cranial cavity (not to be confused with migraines that "migrate" from one side of the head to the other).

INDICATIONS	TREATMENT
You have head pain due to a high fever; you are red and you sweat; you are thirsty	Belladonna 5 CH 2 pillules 3 times a day
You have head pain, a red face, and pulsating temples	Glonoine 5 CH 2 pillules 3 times a day
Your headache diminishes when you are distracted, but it comes back in situations you do not like	Ignatia amara 5 CH 2 pillules 3 times a day
You have a headache due to poor digestion	Antimonium crudum 5 CH 2 pillules 3 times a day
Your headache is due to digestive problems; you are liverish	Lycopodium 5 CH 2 pillules 3 times a day
You have a headache due to poor digestion, with nausea	Ipecac 5 CH 2 pillules 3 times a day
You have a headache due to an injury	Arnica montana 9 CH 2 pillules 3 times a day *combined with* Actaea racemosa 5 CH 2 pillules 3 times a day

INDICATIONS	TREATMENT
Your headache is due to exposure to dry cold or to excessive heat; it is accompanied by sudden fever and anxiety	Aconitum napellus 5 CH 2 pillules 3 times a day
You have a headache before your period and it diminishes when it starts	Folliculinum 9 CH 1 dose on the 14th day of the cycle
You have a headache, and you put on weight before your period, but everything returns to normal when it starts	Bovista 5 CH 2 pillules 3 times a day
Your headache is accompanied by water retention	Natrum sulphuricum 5 CH 2 pillules 3 times a day
You have intermittent acute headaches that feel like a nail in your head	Ignatia amara 5 CH 2 pillules 3 times a day
You have a headache with a sense of melancholy	Sepia 9 CH 2 pillules 3 times a day
Your headache gets worse between 1 and 3 a.m.; it is better with fresh air on your face, even if you are chilly	Arsenicum album 5 CH 2 pillules 3 times a day
Your headache is always worse at night and in damp or stormy weather	Rhododendron 5 CH 2 pillules 3 times a day

INDICATIONS	TREATMENT
For students, headaches that occur after prolonged mental work at the same time as tiredness	Kalium phosphoricum 5 CH 2 pillules 3 times a day
For students, headaches that occur when they shut themselves away and cannot work	Natrum muriaticum 9 CH 2 pillules 3 times a day
For students who are thin and chilly, headaches that are aggravated by the full moon	Silicea 9 CH 2 pillules 3 times a day
Your headache is aggravated by intellectual effort and better when you eat	Anacardium orientale 5 CH 2 pillules 3 times a day

See also: Migraine, page 223.

ADVICE

When you feel a headache coming on, try to go somewhere peaceful. Rest in a quiet room with low light.

ALTITUDE SICKNESS

Discomfort caused by a lack of oxygen at high altitude. You have vertigo, headaches, buzzing in the ears, and palpitations.

INDICATIONS	TREATMENT
In all cases	Coca 5 CH 2 pillules 3 times a day
Altitude sickness gives you nausea	Coca 5 CH 2 pillules 3 times a day *combined with* Cocculus indicus 5 CH 2 pillules 3 times a day

ADVICE

In the most acute cases, supplemental oxygen may be essential.

MOTION SICKNESS

Discomfort with headache and nausea, experienced when you use any kind of transportation (boat, car, or airplane)

INDICATIONS	TREATMENT
You feel better in the fresh air and worse in a confined space; you have nausea and vomiting that worsen in a boat or car	Tabacum 5 CH 2 pillules 3 times a day
Rest makes you better; you feel better in a confined space	Cocculus indicus 5 CH 2 pillules 3 times a day

INDICATIONS	TREATMENT
You feel better when you eat	Petroleum 5 CH 2 pillules 3 times a day
You feel worse before leaving or just after arriving	Ignatia amara 5 CH 2 pillules 3 times a day
You feel worse after drinking alcohol and feel sleepy after meals	Nux vomica 5 CH 2 pillules 3 times a day

Distraction often helps children to forget that they are carsick; provide games, songs, and other activities to occupy them. Arrange things so that the child can see out of the window in the car; looking at a point on the horizon helps to diminish the feeling of discomfort. Do not hesitate to make regular stops so that everyone can stretch their legs and take their mind off things.

BAD CIRCULATION

See: Circulation (problems with), varicose veins, heavy legs, hemorrhoids, page 108.

BAD BREATH

Fetid stench in the mouth.

INDICATIONS	TREATMENT
You have fetid breath; you salivate a lot; you have nausea and a white tongue	Mercurius solubilis 5 CH 2 pillules 3 times a day

INDICATIONS	TREATMENT
You have bad breath with acid eructations and heartburn	Iris versicolor 5 CH 2 pillules 3 times a day Robinia 5 CH 2 pillules 3 times a day
You have bad breath after a heavy meal, and digestion is difficult	Antimonium crudum 5 CH 2 pillules 3 times a day
You have bad breath, you perspire, your skin is unhealthy, and you are extremely chilly	Psorinum 9 CH 2 pillules 3 times a day
Your bad breath is due to a dental infection	Pyrogenium 5 CH 2 pillules 3 times a day *combined with* Calcarea fluorica 5 CH 2 pillules 3 times a day

ADVICE

Avoid tobacco and strong-tasting food, such as garlic; chew gum containing chlorophyll; and take care of your oral hygiene.

MEMORY PROBLEMS

Often temporary incapacity to remember. You are tired or stressed, you have taken medicine such as tranquilizers or sleeping pills, you feel depressed, you drink too much, or you have had a blow to the head, and now you can't remember a name, you don't know where you put something, or you forget the date for something.

INDICATIONS	TREATMENT
For an unruly and agitated child	Mercurius solubilis 5 CH 2 pillules 3 times a day
For a student	Kalium phosphoricum 5 CH 2 pillules 3 times a day
For adults (including older adults)	Phosphoricum acidum 5 CH 2 pillules 3 times a day
You have memory lapses due to stage fright	Gelsemium 5 CH 2 pillules 3 times a day
You have memory lapses due to nervous tiredness	Kalium bromatum 5 CH 2 pillules 3 times a day
You have memory lapses due to general slowing down of your system	Baryta carbonicum 5 CH 2 pillules 3 times a day
You especially have memory lapses between 4 and 8 p.m. (Particularly if you have liver problems)	Lycopodium 5 CH 2 pillules 3 times a day
You have memory lapses due to your lack of self-confidence	Silicea 5 CH 2 pillules 3 times a day
Your memory comes back when you eat	Anacardium orientale 5 CH 2 pillules 3 times a day

ADVICE

Provide your brain, like all of your body, with a healthy and balanced diet. Train your memory by maintaining regular intellectual activity.

MENOPAUSE

End of a woman's ovaries working. You no longer have periods; you suffer from hot flashes and sweating. Your skin becomes dry. You do not absorb calcium as well as you did previously, and your bones become fragile. You sleep less well and have a tendency to become depressed or put on weight.

INDICATIONS	TREATMENT
To combat demineralization	*Combine the three Calcareas:* Calcarea phosphorica 5 CH Calcarea carbonica 5 CH Calcarea fluorica 5 CH 2 pillules 3 times a day *with* Silicea 5 CH 2 pillules 3 times a day
Your last period was painful; the blood was black and formed clots	Secale cornutum 5 CH 2 pillules 3 times a day
To counteract hot flashes when you get them	Belladonna 5 CH 2 pillules 3 times a day
To prevent hot flashes	FSH (follicle stimulating hormone) 4 CH 2 pillules 3 times a day, from the 14th to the 21st day of the cycle
To counteract hot flashes if your temples pulsate	Glonoine 5 CH 2 pillules 3 times a day
You are strong and you sweat a lot	Sulfur 5 CH 2 pillules 3 times a day

INDICATIONS	TREATMENT
You alternate between mental/emotional, and physical problems	Actaea racemosa 7 CH 2 pillules 3 times a day
You suffer from rheumatism and migraines, accompanied by respiratory problems and blotchy skin	Sanguinaria canadensis 5 CH 2 pillules 3 times a day
You have generalized water retention	Natrum sulphuricum 7 CH 2 pillules 3 times a day
The ending of your period is accompanied by chilliness, slight anemia, and skin problems	Graphites 5 CH 2 pillules 3 times a day
You have circulation problems or prolapsed organs; you are depressed and tired from when you wake in the morning	Sepia 9 CH 2 pillules 3 times a day
To manage mental/emotional problems, when they are aggravated by alcohol	Lachesis 9 CH 2 pillules 3 times a day

See also: Excessive appetite, page 78.

ADVICE

At mealtime, avoid food that is too spicy, alcohol, and stimulants like coffee. During the day, wear light, comfortable clothes. Doing relaxation exercises before bedtime and at night, sleep in a room that is not too hot.

MIGRAINE

Headache located on one side of the head. You begin to experience pain above one eye or at one point on the forehead, then you soon have pain all over one side of the head. Any effort becomes painful, as are light and noise. You have pulsating temples and you feel nauseated.

INDICATIONS	TREATMENT
MIGRAINE ON THE RIGHT SIDE	
The migraine starts above the right eye socket	Sanguinaria canadensis 5 CH 2 pillules at the time of the migraine
Your pain is generally located on the right, especially between 4 and 8 p.m.; you can also be peevish	Lycopodium 9 CH 2 pillules 3 times a day *or* 1 dose a week
You have a right-sided migraine accompanied by pain crossing over to the left (left breast, left ovary, left-sided sciatica, and so on)	Actaea racemosa 5 CH 2 pillules 3 times a day
MIGRAINE ON THE LEFT SIDE	
The migraine starts above the left eye socket	Spigelia 5 CH 2 pillules at the time of the migraine
Your pain is generally located on the left; you have circulatory problems	Lachesis 9 CH 2 pillules 3 times a day *or* 1 dose a week

INDICATIONS	TREATMENT
MIGRAINE GOING FROM ONE SIDE TO THE OTHER	
The pain migrates from one side of the head to the other	Lac caninum 9 CH 2 pillules at the time of the migraine
The migraine is difficult to locate; it is aggravated by being in a confined space	Pulsatilla 9 CH 2 pillules at the time of the migraine
The migraine always comes back at the same time	Belladonna 5 CH 2 pillules 3 times a day
The migraine comes on before your period and disappears after it starts	Folliculinum 9 CH 1 dose on the 14th day of the cycle 1 dose on the 21st day of the cycle
The migraine comes back intermittently, alternating with skin problems	Psorinum 9 CH 2 pillules 3 times a day

ADVICE

The migraines are often triggered by the same causes in one person. Try to identify the origin to guard against migraines. If you have not escaped the onset of migraine, stay lying down in a peaceful, dark place.

FUNGAL INFECTION

Infection due to a parasitic fungus. It can cause small lesions on the skin, white deposits if it affects the mouth, or white, irritating discharge when it develops on the vaginal mucous membranes.

INDICATIONS	TREATMENT
Before any treatment, to drain the mucous membranes	Hydrastis 5 CH 2 pillules 3 times a day *combined with* Helonias 5 CH 2 pillules 3 times a day
The discharge is not irritating	Pulsatilla 9 CH 2 pillules 3 times a day
It is a case of *Candida albicans*	Candida albicans 9 CH 2 pillules 3 times a day *combined with* Drainage remedy for vaginal mucous membranes *(See: Complex remedies, page 320)* 20 drops 3 times a day
It is a case of mycosis with ulcerations	Mercurius corrosivus 5 CH 2 pillules 3 times a day

ADVICE

A sample for analysis is indispensable to precisely determine the pathology, so seek medical advice.

NAUSEA, VOMITING

Expulsion of the contents of the stomach through the mouth. You have abdominal pain, heartburn, and nausea, and a sudden spasm to rid yourself of all that is in your stomach.

INDICATIONS	TREATMENT
In all cases	Ipecac 5 CH 2 pillules 3 times a day

INDICATIONS	TREATMENT
The vomiting is better when a hot water bottle placed on your abdomen	Arsenicum album 5 CH 2 pillules 3 times a day
The nausea is better when you eat	Petroleum 5 CH 2 pillules 3 times a day
The vomiting is severe, uncontrollable, clear like water, and aggravated in the evening	Phosphorus 9 CH 1 dose every day for 3 days
Tobacco or the smell of tobacco makes you feel sick	Tabacum 5 CH 2 pillules 3 times a day
The vomiting is accompanied by acid indigestion	Robinia 5 CH 2 pillules 3 times a day
Nausea accompanied by cough	Lobelia inflata 5 CH 2 pillules 3 times a day
For nausea in a pregnant woman	Ipecac 5 CH 2 pillules 3 times a day *combined with* Ignatia amara 5 CH 2 pillules 3 times a day
You become nauseated when you brush your teeth	Sepia 5 CH 2 pillules 3 times a day

ADVICE

In case of serious vomiting, be careful you do not become dehydrated. If you really cannot keep anything down, try decarbonated Coke: stir a glass of very cold Coke vigorously to get rid of all the gas, and then take it 1 teaspoon at a time. That works well for children.

See also: Pregnancy, page 181.

NERVOUSNESS, STRESS

Temporary or chronic state of nervous anxiety in reaction to the difficulties of modern life or to a strong psychological trauma. The stress can be shown in common problems: aggressiveness, depression, psychological conditions, great anxiety, even heart problems.

INDICATIONS	TREATMENT
You are stressed and nervous and tend to have a short fuse	Nux vomica 9 CH 2 pillules 3 times a day
You cannot stay still, and your agitation is calmed by movement	Rhus toxicodendron 5 CH 2 pillules 3 times a day
Your nervousness is aggravated by alcohol	Lachesis 9 CH 2 pillules 3 times a day
Your stress causes incessant agitation of the hands	Kalium bromatum 5 CH 2 pillules 3 times a day
Your stress causes .incessant agitation of the legs	Zincum metallicum 5 CH 2 pillules 3 times a day
You are stressed and would like to have finished everything before you have begun	Argentum nitricum 9 CH 2 pillules 3 times a day
You tremble with nervousness and are worn out	Gelsemium 9 CH 2 pillules 3 times a day

INDICATIONS	TREATMENT
Your nervousness makes you shut down	Natrum muriaticum 9 CH 2 pillules 3 times a day
You have a tendency to avoid company, your nervousness makes you emotional, and you have insomnia	Ambra grisea 9 CH 2 pillules 3 times a day
You find it impossible to express yourself, and this makes you nervous	Staphysagria 9 CH 2 pillules 3 times a day
Your stress and nervousness make you depressed	Sepia 9 CH 2 pillules 3 times a day
You feel nervous, especially between the hours of 4 and 8 p.m.	Lycopodium 9 CH 2 pillules 3 times a day
In the case of an aggressive child who has nightmares and cannot tolerate strong light but asks for a small night light	Stramonium 9 CH 2 pillules 3 times a day
With a child who is worried by their pain, particularly dental	Chamomilla 9 CH 2 pillules 3 times a day
In the case of a child who can't leave anything alone	Tarentula hispana 5 CH 2 pillules 3 times a day

ADVICE

You need to learn to distance yourself from everyday annoyances; what is really important, after all? Remove yourself, from time to time, from the daily routine and go to the movies or go for a walk for an hour. Have a massage, and make time for a few minutes' relaxation every day. Take a relaxing bath and forget about everything for a while. Allow your coffee to get cold without drinking it; you can make a cup of herbal tea later on.

BLOCKED NOSE

When you have a cold, your nose is completely obstructed. You sound like a duck when you talk, cannot blow your nose, and have difficulty breathing. At night, you snore.

INDICATIONS	TREATMENT
Your nose is blocked night and day	Sambucus nigra 5 CH 2 pillules 3 times a day
Your nose is blocked at night and runs during the day	Nux vomica 5 CH 2 pillules 3 times a day
Your nose is blocked at night, and you have problems breathing	Ammonium carbonicum 5 CH 2 pillules 3 times a day
Your nose is blocked in damp weather, after rain or near water (the ocean, a lake, a river)	Dulcamara 5 CH 2 pillules 3 times a day
You have a cold with a dry, wheezy cough; you sneeze	Sticta pulmonaria 5 CH 2 pillules 3 times a day
Your nose is blocked, and you have pain in the frontal sinuses	Cinnabaris 5 CH 2 pillules 3 times a day

Remember the advantages of using saline solution to clear the nostrils. Use very soft handkerchiefs to avoid inflammation of the nostrils. Consider humidifying the rooms in your house, especially the bedrooms.

OBESITY

See: Excess appetite, page 78.

BLACK EYE

You have been hit in the eye, and bruising forms. You have a shiner, a bit painful and not very attractive, but not really dangerous, as the eye itself is not affected.

INDICATIONS	TREATMENT
In all cases	Arnica montana 9 CH
	2 pillules 3 times a day
	combined with
	Ledum palustre 5 CH
	2 pillules 3 times a day

ADVICE

If you do not have a really cold steak, try applying cold compresses or a bag of ice as soon as possible to avoid forming a hematoma. If your eye becomes red, if the cornea is cut, if you think your sight is affected or if you have continuing pain, see an ophthalmologist immediately.

BRITTLE, STAINED, OR DOUBLE NAILS

Your nails are brittle and you cannot get them to grow. They are ridged, soft, thin, double, or have white patches.

INDICATIONS	TREATMENT
Your nails are hard and grow double	Graphites 5 CH 2 pillules 3 times a day
Your nails are soft and marked with white patches	Silicea 5 CH 2 pillules 3 times a day

ADVICE

Fragile nails may be the sign of a poor general state of health, stress, or tiredness. Look for whatever is not right to treat the original cause. You can also try using nail polish with a solidifying base regularly to allow time for them to regenerate.

CHAPTER 4

WHICH REMEDY PROFILE SUITS WHICH PERSONALITY?

Which remedies are made for you?

What is a profile?

THE HOMEOPATHIC PROFILE MAKES IT POSSIBLE TO understand how a person operates and determine their pathological tendencies in order to practice preventive medicine.

It takes account of numerous factors: behavior, physique, and habits. By just seeing a person, shaking their hand (is it soft, firm, clammy, or cold?), observing their face (is it wrinkled, red, pale, or shriveled?), and listening to them speak (are they nervous, exhausted, shy, haughty, gossipy, or reserved?), you can envision the homeopathic personality of each person.

These indications are so many warning signs that make it possible to begin to understand the person better, but they can also sow the seeds of numerous errors of interpretation. This is why homeopathic doctors have traditionally subjected their patients to long questionnaires.

TOOL OF PREVENTIVE MEDICINE

Once determined, the profile makes it possible to foresee the pathological profile of the person. You can imagine how they would react if they got the flu or at the time of giving birth (a Sepia will be more easily affected by "baby blues"), which illnesses may affect them more frequently (an Argentum nitricum will perhaps be subject to stomach ulcers, a Platina will certainly have gynecological problems, and a Staphysagria will surely suffer from suppressed illnesses due to not expressing their problems).

TOOL OF PERSONALIZED MEDICINE

Once the problem is stated, you know from the profile that people who are sick will not react in the same way. Therefore, you can prescribe the remedies that completely match their terrain and their personality, not so much for the illness itself but to improve the everyday life of the person.

There are doctors who even think that one single remedy, the remedy for the profile, would be enough to treat all the conditions that the person may suffer from. But I would not advise using this method as it entails too much risk of error. If you take the wrong path in defining the profile, you get the wrong remedy and leave the person who is ill without any treatment. I prefer using the profile as an indication, valuable but not unique, to guide me as the treatment develops.

In the pages that follow, you will find a description of some of the main profiles. To refine your self-medication, you may try to recognize yourself in one of them. But you may be a combination of two or three of these portraits. It is also very common to change profiles in the course of your life.

You can then verify your first impression by locating yourself on the grid (See pages 250–259). I would guess, however, that only a homeopathic physician could definitively determine your real profile, and that, after long observation.

The main profiles

ARNICA

Traumatic injury, blows, bumps

Daddy Arnica loves physical activity, but no matter how careful he is, he often comes home with new aches and pains. Stiffness, muscle soreness: all his muscles are painful. He would really like to rest, but even his bed seems hard, and so he sleeps badly.

As soon as Mommy Arnica bumps herself (bumps into furniture or a beam that is too low on a staircase), she gets bruises that are painful with the slightest movement. Even when she reads, sitting quietly in the living room, she gets pain in her back and stiffness in her hands.

Miss Arnica has great difficulty recovering from her first disappointment in love: she had an "injury to the heart" from which she suffers as much as the shock experienced by her brother when he heard that he had failed his high school final exams. Mommy Arnica remains traumatized after her little car accident in Daddy's car, while he is very agitated since his lottery ticket won a little gold mine.

ARGENTUM NITRICUM

Always in a hurry

This family is a real buzzing hive, but the people in it are often overtaken by their own activity.

Daddy Argentum Nitricum never has time for anything. His desk is rarely tidy. At a red light, he roars his engine and starts even before the lights turn green. Even in bed, he is in a hurry and can have premature ejaculations.

Mommy Argentum Nitricum is not very patient. She has difficulty, for example, waiting her turn in the doctor's office: she gets up as soon as the practitioner's door opens, even if she has to sit down again to allow an older person who has been waiting for more than 45 minutes to go first. When she enters the consulting room, she takes off her clothes even before she is asked to. She is in such a hurry to leave that she finishes dressing in the hallway. She often puts on her makeup in the car on the way to work in the morning.

The young Argentum Nitricum is always moving around; he moves incessantly and is incapable of doing one thing at a time. He is what you call a hyperactive child. His mind is teeming with ideas; he starts many things, but always wants to have finished before he starts and rarely finishes anything at all.

Daddy Argentum Nitricum cannot help himself from eating at top speed, but then he is often bloated and suffers from aerophagia. He loves sweet food, which doesn't agree with him. He does not want to tell Mommy, but he has a stomach ulcer.

ARSENICUM ALBUM

Well organized

Mommy Arsenicum Album likes the house to be in order: she has organized a methodical form of storage for each thing, and it is out of the question to store pink dust cloths in the same cupboard as blue dust cloths because they are not even used to clean the same glasses. She drinks often, but always in small quantities. She says she is often tired.

Daddy Arsenicum Album, too, is rather meticulous: he might straighten a picture that is crooked ten times over before being satisfied with the result. He often has a fear of death, especially at night between the hours of 1 and 3 a.m. Awakened by a nagging uneasiness, he feels anxious.

The young Arsenicum Album always feels cold. In class, he always sits next to a radiator but chooses one under a window that is always slightly open, because despite feeling chilly, he loves fresh air.

Daddy Arsenicum Album sorts and re-sorts his magnificent collection of coins with careful attention. Otherwise, you see him rarely with money in his hands: he doesn't like to spend without counting.

Mommy Arsenicum Album has visible illnesses alternating with those that cannot be seen. If she has eczema today, she will suffer from bloating tomorrow. And if she has an outbreak of herpes today, she will have asthma tomorrow.

BARYTA CARBONICA

It is no use running

When Mommy Baryta Carbonica begins something, she finishes it, but always in a leisurely way. Time seems not to exist for her.

Miss Baryta Carbonica is slightly chilly, and her periods are often late. She can even miss one or two cycles.

Daddy Baryta Carbonica looks older than he is. He is a bit overweight and suffers from thyroid problems.

The young Baryta Carbonica has difficulty in school. He perseveres but appears not to be suited to intellectual effort.

BRYONIA

Very tense

If he has a pain somewhere, Daddy Bryonia demands bandages: he often wears a knee pad, an abdominal belt, or elbow supports. He always feels better when he rests, wrapped tightly in something.

Mommy Bryonia likes very tight pantyhose, clothing that hugs the body, and bras that are one size too small. She likes to lie down without moving because movements are painful for her, but her mind is always alert.

The young Bryonia can't bear mornings. He has difficulty in getting up and finds this time of day very difficult. He can't stand people brushing against him or caressing him. He is often constipated and always very thirsty; he likes to drink whole bucketfuls.

CALCAREA CARBONICA

Slowly but surely

The baby Calcarea Carbonica is round and jovial, does not cry much, and cuts his teeth quietly. He can sweat profusely on the forehead, leading to eczema and cradle cap. He has a good appetite and may even eat indigestible things (such as chalk).

Daddy Calcarea Carbonica has a strong constitution. He has a build like a rugby player: quite well rounded. He likes eating and drinking well.

Mommy Calcarea Carbonica is placid but tenacious and always finishes what she has started.

The young Calcarea Carbonica is rather slow at school and finds learning difficult, but he is intelligent and organized.

CUPRUM METALLICUM

Cramps

Daddy Cuprum Metallicum is a good runner but rarely wins competitions because he too often has cramps in the middle of the race.

During the night, Mommy Cuprum Metallicum is awakened by very painful cramps.

The Cuprum Metallicum baby often has spasms that make it difficult for him to breathe.

Mommy Cuprum Metallicum cramps were due to her IUD, since it is made of a metal that does not agree with her. She had to have it taken out.

Miss Cuprum Metallicum has become very thin, and the doctor thinks that this is because she was losing too many minerals.

GELSEMIUM

Trembling

Daddy Gelsemium trembles with fever when he has the flu, with a tropical temperature that leaves him completely exhausted.

Before taking an exam, the young Gelsemium has to stay in the bathroom due to diarrhea. When she is eventually able to come out, she does not feel capable of doing or saying anything; she is incapacitated. She trembles like a leaf in the presence of the teacher.

Daddy Gelsemium has Parkinson's disease. It is often feared that he will become dehydrated because he always says he is not thirsty, and he never wants to drink. This could perhaps be also because he is worried about knocking his glass over yet again, due to his tremor.

HYOSCYAMUS NIGER

Hypersensitive

Daddy Hyoscyamus Niger does not like noises that are too loud or odors that are too strong, and he likes light even less. His reaction to dazzling light can make him seem crazy.

Mommy Hyoscyamus Niger is of a very delicately sensitive disposition. She coughs when she lies down.

Daddy Hyoscyamus Niger has lost awareness of his body. He is no longer fully aware of what he is doing and can sometimes appear naked in front of everyone. He is delirious and often has nightmares.

IGNATIA AMARA

Paradoxical

Mommy Ignatia Amara is pregnant. She used to love coffee but can no longer tolerate it, but she craves strawberries at 4 a.m. on Christmas. She suffers from very specifically located headaches in the middle of the skull.

Miss Ignatia Amara is subject to tetany. She even suffers slightly from panic disorder. She likes distractions, which always improve her condition, but boredom aggravates her symptoms, as does the neighbor whom she cannot bear and who is pursuing her. She only has to see him to develop a headache. Even though she smokes, she is very put out by this young man smoking, which invariably makes her cough. But there is no risk that she will discourage him any time soon; it is because she is unpredictable that he is so attracted by her.

Daddy Ignatia Amara will happily devour sauerkraut in the company of Mommy, whom he still loves with the love of a young man, and would even take more. But he could not eat yogurt with his mother-in-law watching, as she gets on his nerves.

LACHESIS

Loquacious

Mommy Lachesis talks a lot. Alcohol does not agree with her. She has vein problems, but always feels better when her period starts or when she has a sauna session, during which she perspires a great deal.

Daddy Lachesis cannot tolerate a belt or tie or anything else that is too tight. At night he often dreams of death. He has liver problems and always gets left-sided migraines.

Mommy Lachesis has a very red complexion. She has difficulty with menopause. She has bruises all over, even without injuring herself: they appear spontaneously, and she always wonders how. She often thinks that people are saying nasty things about her, and this makes her rather distrustful.

LYCOPODIUM

Rather bossy

If Mommy Lycopodium can sometimes appear overbearing, it is because she is a bit bossy and very determined.

Mommy Lycopodium always has problems on the right side: she often has sciatica or sore throats, always on the right side. She generally feels worse between the hours of 4 and 8 p.m.

The young Lycopodium looks older than he is. At the age of twenty he already has some white hair. His memory lapses cause him problems with studying. Daddy Lycopodium often has eyes that are bigger than his stomach. He frequently orders two or three things in a restaurant but feels bloated after the first few mouthfuls, to the point where he has to loosen his belt. He is bossy, and his bad temper can hide a lack of self-confidence.

Daddy Lycopodium always complains about his liver problems.

MERCURIUS SOLUBILIS

Often ill

The young Mercurius Solubilis often develops sore throats, and his nose is often blocked. With the slightest health problem, he generally goes through the same phases: inflammation, suppuration, ulceration. He is not very good at school but is the leader of the local gang.

Mommy Mercurius Solubilis produces a lot of saliva. She has breath that smells stale and is accompanied by a white tongue. She also has kidney problems.

Miss Mercurius Solubilis often does not sleep well. She is subject to phases of excitement followed by depression.

Daddy Mercurius Solubilis has been subject to mercury inhalation. He has many dental amalgam fillings and has profuse saliva. On his white tongue you can see the imprint of his teeth appearing.

NATRUM MURIATICUM

Rather reserved

Miss Natrum Muriaticum is in the middle of an adolescent crisis. She shuts herself in her room and does not say anything.

Daddy Natrum Muriaticum also does not like talking about himself, particularly to the doctor. He often gets outbreaks of herpes and is always more or less constipated. He is usually very thirsty, with a dry mouth and chapped, even fissured lips, and he cannot stop himself from eating very salty food.

Mommy Natrum Muriaticum always looks rather sad and doesn't like being consoled. During her persistent flu, she has lost a lot of minerals and feels dried out. As a result, the upper half of her body has grown thin, the lower half swollen, with a tendency toward cellulite. She gets a bit depressed at night and dreams of burglars and dogs.

As for the young Natrum Muriaticum, he gets tired easily at school. He has memory problems and difficulty learning his lessons. As a result, he loses confidence in himself. Instead of playing with the others during recess, he prefers to stay on his own in a corner. School breaks do not bring him any respite: this year, he has to visit his aunt who lives near the ocean. Everyone says that he will really enjoy himself at the beach, but he knows that this is not the case. He never feels well at the beach.

NUX VOMICA

Hyperactive and exhausted

He is a modern man—a hyperactive, exhausted company director—and works too hard. He has quite a short fuse and sometimes is a little aggressive, but his associates know that his angry outbursts are not followed up and don't last long. He quickly forgets that he was angry.

He goes from one business lunch to another and likes drinking a glass or two, but after that he is sleepy in the early afternoon. He would love to have a little siesta, but when?

To counteract feeling under par, he drinks gallons of coffee, chain-smokes, and sometimes even resorts to illicit substances. He eats very spicy food and never skimps on the pepper and salt. However much these habits help him to cope, they are not without disadvantages: he suffers from hemorrhoids and his bowel function constantly fluctuates between constipation and diarrhea. By polluting his own system in this way, he only aggravates his physical state and his tension. To make matters worse, he doesn't manage to do any physical activity.

In the evening, he falls asleep in front of the television, but once in bed, he can never sleep: he goes over the events of the day and regularly pays for this with insomnia. He eventually drifts off at about 6 a.m., just before the alarm rings. So, feeling tired, he uses some stimulants, sets off again with his hectic lifestyle, and becomes the ideal candidate for stomach ulcers, a celibate life, or divorce.

PHOSPHORUS

Enthusiastic

Daddy Phosphorus is always very fit and full of energy during the day, but he doesn't like nightfall. His voice gets hoarse, and he never feels well at dusk.

The young Phosphorus is a tall adolescent who is a bit gangly and gives the impression of having grown too fast. He flares up quickly and always takes part in many projects, which rapidly become passions, but he passes as quickly from one to the next. He is impulsive and fiery, and there he is, always ready to confront the world. His little brother, tall for his age, has a stoop. He already has breathing difficulties due to having compressed his lungs. He often has nosebleeds, is afraid of storms, and never feels secure at night. He has had hepatitis.

Mommy Phosphorus is often tired. Her diarrhea and her periods, always very profuse, don't help at all.

PLATINA

Arrogant and haughty

Mr. Platina easily feels superior to others and crushes them with his arrogance, even if it is not always justified. He is master of his own universe, and he would also like to dominate the larger universe.

Mrs. Platina may appear rather haughty. Concerned about her image and social standing, she always wears fine clothes—sometimes a little eccentric but always sought after—very valuable jewelry, and careful makeup. She rarely finds a partner who she thinks is good enough for her. She is very often sexually excited.

PULSATILLA

Tender and gentle

Miss Pulsatilla is very kind and a bit shy and has a pleasant personality. Her first period started a bit later than her friends' did, and her periods are always very short. She already has blue-veined marbling on her ankles, like the women who are going to have circulation problems, but long walks in the fresh air make her feel good.

Her little sister tends to get sore throats but without a high fever. Her temperature varies but stays at around 100°F. She always clings to her comforting stuffed animal, without which she cannot sleep. In the case of real heartbreak, Mini Pulsatilla goes from crying to laughing in an instant if she likes the person who is consoling her.

Mommy Pulsatilla is tender and sensitive. Moreover, there is nothing irritating about her: when she has a cold, the discharge from her nose or her eyes is clear and soft; when she has a vaginal discharge, it is never irritating. She is a little chilly; her hands, feet, and nose are cold. But she does not necessarily like overheated places. She is vulnerable and a little frightened of men, except in Daddy's case, because she loves him.

RHUS TOXICODENDRON

They move about

Daddy Rhus Toxicodendron moves about all the time, and he likes that. He says that movement helps him. So, he moves constantly, even at night; he tosses and turns in his sleep. Sometimes he even dreams of moving to another home.

Mommy Rhus Toxicodendron is a bit slow to get going in the morning, but then she is agitated the whole day long like a little working ant, which leaves her completely exhausted in the evening. Miss Rhus Toxicodendron has alternating nerve pain and skin problems, especially eruptions of little vesicles, like shingles or herpes.

Daddy Rhus Toxicodendron does not like the fall. This hellish season always brings its share of rain and humidity, which bring back his rheumatism. And Mommy makes him rest again: she has really never understood that rest doesn't help him at all.

SEPIA

Sad

Daddy Sepia never feels as well as when he is doing energetic physical activity. But most often, he puts on a somber, sad expression. He often wears black and has a tendency to turn in on himself. He is subject to depression with a kind of fatalistic resignation.

Mommy Sepia is pregnant. Her pregnancy is going well, in spite of the patches on her face. She picks up urinary tract infections and thinks that her belly weighs a ton. After the birth of her first child, she suffers from postpartum depression and feels like crying all the time. Mommy Sepia likes vinegar, pickles, and acidic foods. She is subject to hemorrhoids, varicose veins, and urinary problems.

SILICEA

Frail and intelligent

Mommy Silicea is very frail. She is intelligent and succeeds very well in her career. However, she has a tendency to underestimate herself and always remains a bit reserved.

Since his last sore throat, Daddy Silicea feels tired. He is demineralized and has lost a lot of weight. He feels cold often. His hands and feet are cold, even though his feet still sweat a lot.

The young Silicea is constantly sick. As his teacher says, he catches anything that is going around and will catch the first virus that comes along. The result of this is that he gets infection after infection and now has chronic discharges. It is not really surprising that he is always tired.

STAPHYSAGRIA

Subdued

Daddy Staphysagria does not talk much, not about his problems, anyway. He hedges his bets, and he somatizes. When he is really at his wits' end, sometimes he allows himself to slam a door shut.

That Mommy Staphysagria's boss is abusively domineering is well known. Often she would like to shout out her indignation, but nothing comes out. As a result, she becomes a bit depressed and no longer counts the little spots that are appearing on her face.

The young Staphysagria is subjected to his teacher's wrath, even though the ringleader is not him but the little boy who sits right next to him in class. When he puts up his hand to answer, the teacher never calls on him. And then she gives him a bad grade on his oral exam. So much injustice makes him vomit, in the strict sense of the term, but he does not manage to protest.

SULFUR

Jovial

Daddy Sulfur is a happy person. He is always joyful and communicates his good humor to everyone. He is hale and hearty and doesn't like wearing a tie; furthermore, he does not worry much about being meticulous about what he wears. He often feels hot and sweats a lot. There is no reason for that to change. Moreover, the doctor, when renewing his prescription for hypertension, advises him not to use antiperspirants. "Eliminations are good for you," he says.

Mommy Sulfur is intelligent and happy. There is no problem with her. She is a little well-padded but she lives well. She says that she is never ill. She likes eating and drinking well. Although she never does any physical exercise, she is, nevertheless, a bit tired, with frequent digestive difficulties, but never at the same time as her skin problems.

Daddy Sulfur loves life: he has always loved laughter, eating, drinking, making love, and living in general. When he goes to sleep, he always wants to be on the cooler side of the bed and takes his feet out from under the covers. In the morning, however, like a young boy, he begrudgingly takes a shower: it will, without fail, start his itching again.

THUJA OCCIDENTALIS

Aquaphobe

Daddy Thuja doesn't like water; his rheumatism comes back every time it rains. He was very sick as a child. Today, he is absolutely fine, but he feels poisoned by all the medicines, antibiotics, and corticosteroids that he has had to take for years. His proneness to depression is worse when the climate is damp.

The young Thuja picks up warts. He has just been vaccinated against tetanus and isn't recovering from it very well.

Mommy Thuja, who is subject to water retention, has a bit of cellulite. Sometimes, obsessive thoughts keep her from sleeping.

What is your profile?

Do you recognize some of your personality traits in any of these profiles? Confirm your impression by taking this quick test.

INSTRUCTIONS

In the tables on the following pages, check all the boxes that are appropriate for you. For example, if you are calm and have a quiet personality, check all the boxes in the "I am calm" row that are marked with a + symbol. if you have headaches, check the ones from which you suffer the most; and so on. Then add up the number of boxes checked per column (one profile per column). The maximum total corresponds to your profile. If you get equal scores, choose the common characteristics and the two corresponding remedies to treat yourself.

MEANING OF SYMBOLS	
+	yes, often
+/–	sometimes, from time to time
<	aggravated by
>	better from

	ARGENTUM NITRICUM	ARSENICUM ALBUM	BARYTA CARBONICA	IGNATIA AMARA	LACHESIS	LYCOPODIUM	MERCURIUS SOLUBILIS	NATRUM MURIATICUM
I AM ACTIVE, AGITATED	+	+		+	+		+	
I AM CALM			+					+
I AM AGGRESSIVE				+	+	+	+	
I AM TIRED		+	+	+/–	+/–	+	+/–	+
I HAVE MEMORY PROBLEMS	+		+		+	+/–	+/–	+
I SLEEP BADLY	+	+		+/–	+		+	+/–
I FEEL BETTER IN THE WARM	+/–	+	+	+/–				
I FEEL BETTER IN THE COLD					+			
I FEEL BETTER IN THE FRESH AIR		+		+	+	+		+
I FEEL WORSE WITH HEAT					+	+	+	
I FEEL WORSE WITH COLD	+	+	+			+	+	

NUX VOMICA	PHOSPHORUS	PLATINA	PULSATILLA	SEPIA	SILICEA	STAPHYSAGRIA	SULFUR	THUJA OCCIDENTALIS
+	+	+				+	+	
			+	+	+			+
+		+				+		
+	+/-	+	+/-	+	+	+		+
	+/-				+	+		
+	+/-	+		+/-		+		+
					+			
							+	
			+				+	
							+	
+			+		+			

	ARGENTUM NITRICUM	ARSENICUM ALBUM	BARYTA CARBONICA	IGNATIA AMARA	LACHESIS	LYCOPODIUM	MERCURIUS SOLUBILIS	NATRUM MURIATICUM
I FEEL WORSE WHEN IT IS DAMP		+/-						
I FEEL BETTER WHEN I AM MOVING		+/-			+/-			
I FEEL BETTER WHEN I AM RESTING			+					
I HAVE HEADACHES	+ due to sweets	+/-		+	+ on the left	+ on the right	+/- in the evening	+
I HAVE MIGRAINES	+ due to sweets			+	+ on the left	+ on the right	+/- in the evening	+
I HAVE BLOATING	+ due to sweets	+ with burning sensations		+/- > from distraction	+/-	-+ below the navel	+/-	
I HAVE DIARRHEA	+ due to sweets	+ burning		+/- > from distraction	+ which makes me feel better	+/- with gas	+ with greenish mucus	
I AM CONSTIPATED				+/- > from distraction		+/-		+
I HAVE HEARTBURN	+ due to sweets	+/- > hot water bottle		+/- > from distraction		+/-	+/-	
TOTAL								

NUX VOMICA	PHOSPHORUS	PLATINA	PULSATILLA	SEPIA	SILICEA	STAPHYSAGRIA	SULFUR	THUJA OCCIDENTALIS
								+
+			slowly	quickly			+	
+					+			
+ after meals	+/– in the evening	+	+ in a warm room	+	+ in the cold on exertion	+	+ from heat	+ with fixed ideas
+/– after meals	+/– in the evening	+	+ in a warm room	hepatic		+	+ from heat	+
+/– after meals								
	+/–		+/–	+/–			+ at 5 a.m.	morning
+		traveling	+/–	+/–	+			
+/–						+/–	+/–	

	ARGENTUM NITRICUM	ARSENICUM ALBUM	BARYTA CARBONICA	IGNATIA AMARA	LACHESIS	LYCOPODIUM	MERCURIUS SOLUBILIS	NATRUM MURIATICUM
I HAVE ULCERATIONS	+ due to sweets	+/- > hot water bottle		+/- > distraction	+/-		+/-	+/- and dry skin
I HAVE VARICOSE VEINS					+	+/-		+/- and dry skin
I HAVE HEMORRHOIDS	+ Fissured due to sweets	+/- > heat		+/-	+/-	+/-	+/-	+/- and dry mucous membranes
I HAVE SPASMS	+/- due to sweets	+/-		+	+	+/- with flatulence	+ at night	
I HAVE ASTHMA OR RESPIRATORY PROBLEMS	+ due to sweets	+ with anxiety	+/-	+	+> anything tight	+ < from 4 to 8 p.m.	+/- < at night	+/- < by the ocean
I OFTEN HAVE SORE THROATS	+ due to sweets	+ > hot drinks	+ gland	+/- < boredom	on the left	on the right	+ white	+/- with herpes
I OFTEN HAVE HERPES		+/-			+/- on the left	+/- on the right		+ dry lips
I PERSPIRE A LOT			+/-				+	+
I HAVE PROFUSE SALIVA							+	
I FEEL WORSE WHEN I EAT SWEETS	+			+/-		+/-		

NUX VOMICA	PHOSPHORUS	PLATINA	PULSATILLA	SEPIA	SILICEA	STAPHYSAGRIA	SULFUR	THUJA OCCIDENTALIS
+/–	+/–	+				+/–	+/–	
+			+ ankles marbled with blue veins	+			+/–	+/–
+	+/–	+/–	+	+			+/– red	
+	+/–	+	+/–	+		+	+/–	
+ < after meals	+ < in the evening	+/–	+ < from fresh air	+/–	+ immuno-deficient	+ < vexation	+/– > from cold	+ < medicines and humidity
	hoarse in the evening		+/–	before periods	+/–	+ < vexation	+/– red	
	+/–						+/– red	
					feet		+	+
		+/–	+/–					+/–
+/–							+/–	

	ARGENTUM NITRICUM	ARSENICUM ALBUM	BARYTA CARBONICA	IGNATIA AMARA	LACHESIS	LYCOPODIUM	MERCURIUS SOLUBILIS	NATRUM MURIATICUM
I FEEL WORSE WHEN I EAT SALTY								+
I FEEL WORSE WHEN I EAT ACIDIC FOOD				+/−				
I FEEL WORSE WHEN I EAT . . .				with someone I don't like	when wearing something tight	beer oysters		by the ocean
I OFTEN FEEL THIRSTY		+ in small quantities		+/−	+ alcohol		+ and I have a lot of saliva	+
TOTAL								

NUX VOMICA	PHOSPHORUS	PLATINA	PULSATILLA	SEPIA	SILICEA	STAPHYSAGRIA	SULFUR	THUJA OCCIDENTALIS
								+
+		.		+				
spicy	when I drink		butter, greasy	vinegar				
+ alcohol			never thirsty				+	

	ARGENTUM NITRICUM	ARSENICUM ALBUM	BARYTA CARBONICA	IGNATIA AMARA	LACHESIS	LYCOPODIUM	MERCURIUS SOLUBILIS	NATRUM MURIATICUM
I HAVE LIVER PROBLEMS	+/– due to stress	+	+/–	+/– paradoxical	+ alcohol	+		
I FEEL WORSE BY THE OCEAN								+
I HAVE VERTIGO	+ from heights			+/–	+/–	hepatic	+	
I FEEL BETTER WHEN I AM DISTRACTED				+				
I FEEL BETTER WITH CONSOLATION								
I FEEL WORSE WITH CONSOLATION				+/–				+
I TALK A LOT					+			
I DO NOT TALK MUCH				+/–		+		+
THE TIME WHEN ALL MY SYMPTOMS GET WORSE	at night	1 to 3 a.m.			morning	4 to 8 p.m.	at night	9 to 11 a.m.
TOTAL								

NUX VOMICA	PHOSPHORUS	PLATINA	PULSATILLA	SEPIA	SILICEA	STAPHYSAGRIA	SULFUR	THUJA OCCIDENTALIS
+ sedentary life	+		< rich foods	+		+/– < vexation	+/– > eliminations	+ vaccines, medicines
+/–								+
			with someone I like			+		
			+		with reassurance			
				+				
	+/–	+ haughty					+	
	+/–		+	+		+		
sleepiness after meals	evening and dusk	at night		11 a.m.	full moon	indignation	6 a.m.	3 to 4 a.m.

CHAPTER 5

WHICH REMEDIES DO YOU NEED IN YOUR PHARMACY?

Your personalized basic remedy kit.

CREATE A HOMEOPATHIC PHARMACY FOR EACH person. Adapt yours to your family's circumstances, your job, and your general activities.

Select the kit that suits you best from this list and add specific remedies for your needs to the basic kit. In this way, your pharmacy will correspond to your personality and needs.

Before taking any remedies, refer to chapter 3, "Selecting Remedies: Which One for Which Symptom?," page 45, to determine the indications and ideal doses for your case.

HOMEOPATHY

Basic remedy kit

A small number of essential remedies that are useful for everyone:

- 🐝 Aconitum napellus 5 CH: for sudden, high fevers and serious conditions, especially when they are caused by dry cold or by heatstroke and are accompanied by anxiety.

- 🐝 Apis mellifica 5 CH: for insect stings, sunstroke, edema, and swelling with inflammation, when they are better with cold and you are not thirsty.

- 🐝 Arnica montana 9 CH: for physical injury and shock.

- 🐝 Arsenicum album 7 CH: for food poisoning, eczema, and asthma, when they are better with heat, and for extreme, manic anxiety.

- 🐝 Belladonna 5 CH: for burns, inflammation, fever, and pain with redness.

- 🐝 Calendula mother tincture: for wounds and skin conditions (homeopathic Mercurochrome) and mouthwash.

- 🐝 China rubra 5 CH: for all loss of body fluids (bleeding, diarrhea, vomiting, perspiration, ejaculation) followed by great fatigue, and an antidote to quinine.

- 🐝 Gelsemium 9 CH: for anxiety and stage fright with inhibition.

- 🐝 Ignatia amara 9 CH: for situational anxiety, tetany, psychological problems that develop into physical symptoms, and paradoxical manifestations of different conditions.

- Mercurius solubilis 9 CH: for white sore throats, poisoning with heavy metals, and excessive salivation with bad breath.

- Nux vomica 5 CH: for digestive problems after a good meal, abuse of alcohol, and to detoxify.

- Thuja occidentalis 5 CH: for warts and all damage from something external to the system: vaccinations, antibiotics, or cortisone.

Emergency remedy kit

Add to the basic remedy kit:

- Phosphorus 5 CH: for small hemorrhages.

- Veratrum album 5 CH: for loss of consciousness and general weakness.

Kit for babies

Add to the basic remedy kit:

- Chamomilla 9 CH: for teething with diarrhea and irritation.

- Ferrum phosphoricum 5 CH in combination with Mercurius dulcis 5 CH: for otitis.

- Stramonium 9 CH: for nightmares and distress in babies.

Kit for infants

Add to the basic remedy kit:

- Antimonium crudum 9 CH: for greedy children.

- Colocynthis 9 CH: for anger or stress that causes abdominal pain.

- Staphysagria 9 CH: for children who have psychosomatic problems due to timidity and cannot speak about their problems.

Kit for schoolchildren

Add to the basic remedy kit:

- Calcarea carbonicum 9 CH: for a child who is rather heavy and flabby.

- Calcarea phosphorica 9 CH: for too rapid growth.

- Magnesia phosphorica 9 CH: for abdominal pain.

- Natrum muriaticum 9 CH: for a child who sits in their room and does not say anything.

Kit for students

Add to the basic remedy kit:

- Anacardium orientale 9 CH: for the student who compensates for mental fatigue by snacking.

- Gelsemium: for stage fright and anxiety before exams with inability to think.

Pregnancy kit

Add to the basic remedy kit:

- Actaea racemosa 5 CH combined with Caulophyllum 5 CH: to dilate the cervix at the moment of giving birth.

- Colocynthis 5 CH: for spasms and contractions.

- Ipecac 5 CH: for nausea.

- Kalium phosphoricum 9 CH: for fatigue in the second trimester.

- Silicea 9 CH: for demineralization accompanied by lack of self-confidence.

Kit for sports injuries

Add to the basic remedy kit:

- Bryonia 5 CH: for the joints and for pain that is better with immobilization.

- Rhus toxicodendron 5 CH: for pain that is better with movement.

- Ruta graveolens 5 CH: for tendonitis.

Kit for the stressed CEO

Add to the basic remedy kit (making sure that you never forget Nux vomica 5 CH):

- Antimonium crudum 9 CH: for people who compensate for stress by snacking and smoking.

- Argentum nitricum 9 CH: for people who are overworked and never have time to finish what they have started.

Kit for senior citizens

Add to the basic remedy kit:

- Actaea racemosa 9 CH: for senior citizens who have alternating psychological and physical problems.

- Arsenicum album 9 CH: for anxiety and fear of death.

- Baryta carbonicum 9 CH: for exhaustion and weakness, in case of hypertension.

- Calcarea carbonica 9 CH, Calcarea phosphorica 9 CH, Calcarea fluorica 9 CH, and Silica 9 CH: for demineralization.

- Hyoscyamus niger 9 CH: for delusional behavior with exhibitionism.

- Lachesis 9 CH: for anxious, menopausal women with insomnia and who talk a great deal.

- Ledum palustre 5 CH: for pain that is better with cold.

- Symphytum 9 CH: to help rebuild bone after a fracture.

Kit for summer

Add to the basic remedy kit:

- Dulcamara 5 CH: for all disorders and pain triggered by damp.

- Phosphorus 5 CH combined with China rubra 5 CH and Arsenicum album 5 CH: for diarrhea.

Kit for winter

Add to the basic remedy kit:

- Dulcamara 5 CH: for all disorders and pain triggered by damp.

- Serum Yersin 5 CH: for the flu and winter pathologies.

Travel remedy kit

Add to the basic remedy kit:

- Cocculus indicus 5 CH: for travel sickness that is better with air in a confined space and with rest.

- Petroleum 5 CH: for travel sickness aggravated by the smell of gasoline but improved with eating.

- Tabacum 5 CH: for travel sickness that is better with fresh air.

- Veratrum album 5 CH: for loss of consciousness and general weakness.

Kit for tropical countries

Add to the basic remedy kit:

- Baptisia tinctoria 9 CH: for diarrhea that triggers anguish and delirium.

- Ledum palustre 5 CH: for mosquito bites.

- Phosphorus 5 CH: for diarrhea and hemorrhages.

- Rhododendron 5 CH: for disorders and pain triggered by warm damp.

- Veratrum album 5 CH: for loss of consciousness and general weakness.

Dental kit

Add to the basic remedy kit:

- Borax 5 CH: for thrush.

- Chamomilla 9 CH: for pain accompanied by vexation and diarrhea.

- Cina 5 CH: for bruxism due to worms.

- Hepar sulphur 5 CH: to accelerate removal of pus from an abscess.

- Hepar sulphur 15 CH: to dry up pus from an abscess.

- Hypericum perforatum 5 CH: for pain along the nerve path.

- Kreosotum 5 CH: for black teeth and bad breath.

- Ledum palustre 5 CH: for trauma after dental extraction when the pain is better with application of ice.

- Pyrogenium 5 CH: for infections.

- Silicea 9 CH: for chronic infections and demineralization.

- Staphysagria 5 CH: for scarring after surgery.

- Symphytum 9 CH: to help rebuild bone after a fracture.

- Vaccinotoxinum 9 CH in combination with Rhus toxicodendron 5 CH: for labial herpes.

Kit for animals

Add to the basic remedy kit:

- Bryonia 5 CH: for pain that is better with rest and pressure, aggravated by movement, and accompanied by great thirst.

- Cina 5 CH: for worm infestations.

- Hepar sulphur 5 CH: to accelerate removal of pus from an abscess.

- Hepar sulphur 15 CH: to dry up pus from an abscess.

* Hypericum perforatum 5 CH: for puncture wounds (thorns, pointed objects).

* Ledum palustre 5 CH in combination with Apis mellifica 5 CH: for tick or insect bites.

* Phosphorus 5 CH: for cuts and animal bites.

* Pyrogenium 5 CH: for infections.

* Staphysagria 9 CH: for animals distressed by a master who treats them too harshly or by a traumatic event.

* Symphytum 9 CH: to help rebuild bone after a fracture.

CHAPTER 6

THE REMEDIES

The main homeopathic remedies and their indications.

Aconitum napellus	Very high fever (104°F or higher) due to exposure to cold; dry, without perspiration
	Sunstroke
	Sudden headache accompanied by anxiety
	Excitability or panic (fear of death) with redness and palpitations in asthenic people

REMEDY NAME	INDICATIONS
Actaea racemosa	ᵉ𝒷 Painful periods, if the pain is even more intense during periods ᵉ𝒷 Painful breasts during periods ᵉ𝒷 Regulation of labor while giving birth ᵉ𝒷 Cervical pain (in this case combine with Arnica montana) ᵉ𝒷 Cramps (in this case combine with Cuprum metallicum) ᵉ𝒷 Migraine on the right side ᵉ𝒷 You talk a lot, going off in all directions ᵉ𝒷 Alternating mental/emotional and physical pain; when the person feels physically well, it is the mental/emotional side that has broken down and vice versa
Actaea spicata	ᵉ𝒷 Rheumatism with deformity of small joints ᵉ𝒷 Pain in wrists, hands, and fingers ᵉ𝒷 Eczema on the hands
Aesculus hippocastanum	ᵉ𝒷 Congestive hemorrhoids (large and red) ᵉ𝒷 Varicose veins

REMEDY NAME	INDICATIONS
Aethusa cynapium	⬥ Intolerance of breast milk ⬥ Gastroenteritis of newborn ⬥ Dehydration
Agaricus muscarius	⬥ Twitching of the face ⬥ Senile tremor ⬥ Some Parkinson's problems ⬥ Eye twitching ⬥ Chilblains ⬥ Alcohol poisoning
Allium cepa	⬥ Cold and sneezing aggravated by a warm room ⬥ Watery, irritating nasal discharge
Aloe	⬥ Weeping hemorrhoids ⬥ Acute burning diarrhea ⬥ Fecal incontinence (stained underwear)
Alumina	⬥ Constipation ⬥ Diminished bowel function ⬥ Dryness of the mouth and skin ⬥ Dehydration

REMEDY NAME	INDICATIONS
Ambra grisea	Stage fright
	Emotional reactions, frequently bursting into tears
	Nervousness, stress
	Insomnia
Ammonium carbonicum	Rhinopharyngitis
	Blocked nose
	Asthma, cough in the middle of the night
	Bronchial congestion
	Respiratory difficulties
Anacardium orientale	Eczema, skin problems
	When the symptoms are better when eating
	Mental fatigue, memory problems
	Anxiety
	Headache
	Stomach pain
	Sensation of hunger that causes aggression, excessive appetite
	Obesity

REMEDY NAME	INDICATIONS
Anagallis arvensis	🙲 Skin diseases on the hands or feet
Antimonium crudum	*When the symptoms are accompanied by a white tongue* 🙲 Indigestion after eating to excess 🙲 Warts 🙲 Impetigo
Antimonium tartaricum	*When the symptoms are accompanied by a white tongue* 🙲 Expectoration difficult, better after expulsion 🙲 Bronchitis 🙲 Asthma

REMEDY NAME	INDICATIONS
Apis mellifica	◦ Conjunctivitis ◦ Rose pink edema better with cold applications (compresses, bags of ice) *When the symptoms are accompanied by burning, swollen edema, and the patient passes little or no urine* ◦ Insect bite/sting ◦ Sunburn ◦ Superficial burn ◦ Urticaria ◦ Skin allergy
Aralia racemosa	◦ Asthma at the beginning of the night ◦ Cough that is triggered by lying down ◦ Rhinitis with irritating discharge aggravated by cold

REMEDY NAME	INDICATIONS
Argentum nitricum	*The remedy for people who are in a hurry and who would like to have finished before having begun* 🐑 Jittery with anticipation 🐑 Headache, diarrhea, bloating, stomach pain sometimes with ulceration, when these symptoms are due to emotions or to eating sweet foods 🐑 Sore throat 🐑 Laryngitis
Arnica montana	🐑 Blow, shock, trauma 🐑 Hematoma, bruise 🐑 Bruising 🐑 Muscle soreness (with the flu, exercise injuries, after moving house); even the bed seems too hard 🐑 To prevent muscle soreness before skiing or a session of physical activity 🐑 Mental/emotional shock (after a death, an accident)

REMEDY NAME	INDICATIONS
Arsenicum album	✤ Gastroenteritis due to food poisoning with nausea, vomiting, diarrhea, or abdominal burning sensations, and when the symptoms are better with the application of heat (from a hot water bottle, for example) in people who feel chilly
	✤ Cystitis
	✤ Headache (better in the fresh air)
	✤ Asthma (worse between 1 and 3 a.m.) in a person who is anxious, asthenic, and agitated
	✤ Coryza
	✤ The eczema is dry and burning and better with heat
Arum triphyllum	✤ Painful laryngitis affecting the voice
	✤ Dry, bleeding lips after biting them
Asafoetida	✤ Aerophagia with general flatulence
	✤ Spasms with chest pain
	✤ Acid reflux, regurgitation

REMEDY NAME	INDICATIONS
Aurum metallicum	*When the person has a coppery red face*
	🙠 Depression, sometimes with a suicide attempt (in this case it is essential to see a doctor)
	🙠 Infection of the bones of the ears and nose
Aviaire	🙠 Otitis
	🙠 Bronchitis
	🙠 Bronchiolitis
	🙠 Asthma
	🙠 Following a BCG vaccination (if there is fever, cough, otitis, or any other ear, nose, and throat condition)
Badiaga	🙠 Bouts of asthmatic coughing; coughing spasms
	🙠 Laryngitis
	🙠 Abundant watery discharge (runny nose)
	🙠 Sexual breakdown, impotence
Baptisia tinctoria	🙠 Gastroenteritis with mental/ emotional disorders
	🙠 Gastric flu with pain in the eyes
	🙠 Pharyngitis

REMEDY NAME	INDICATIONS
Baryta carbonica	⁀ Tonsillitis ⁀ Sore throat ⁀ General slowing down, physically, mentally, and hormonally (delayed development, mental slowness, behind with school work, periods late or absent)
Belladonna	⁀ Acute inflammations (rhinopharyngitis, sore throat, otitis) with fever of 100–102°F and perspiration, especially in children ⁀ Febrile delirium with nightmares ⁀ Hot flashes in menopause ⁀ Superficial burns that are hot, red, and painful (sunstroke, initial stage of finger or toe infection, and the like)
Benzoicum acidum	⁀ Cystitis ⁀ Gout attack with inflammation of small joints (such as toes)
Berberis vulgaris	⁀ Kidney and liver drainage (take in combination with other hepatic drainage: Solidago, Taraxacum) ⁀ Urinary insufficiency ⁀ Eczema

REMEDY NAME	INDICATIONS
Blatta orientalis	Acute asthma attack
	Bronchitis
	Bronchiolitis
	Cough
	Allergy to house dust, dust mites, and the like.
Borax	Mouth sores; canker sores
	Vertigo
Bovista	Very heavy periods, sometimes with diarrhea
	Premenstrual syndrome (putting on weight, swelling of breasts with periods)
	Bleeding mid-cycle, at the time of ovulation
	Headache with sensation of the head enlarging
	Generalized water retention, swelling of fingers
Bromum	Respiratory difficulties that are better at sea
	Asthma that is better at sea and worse once returning to land
	Cough
	Laryngitis

REMEDY NAME	INDICATIONS
Bryonia	*When the person is thirsty for large quantities of water*
	✿ The flu, if the person feels better in bed, without moving and with complete rest and pressure on painful parts (head, thorax)
	✿ Bronchitis, tracheitis that is better with rest and not moving
	✿ Dry, painful cough, better with pressure on the thorax
Cactus grandiflorus	✿ Angina pectoris, the feeling of constriction in the chest (if the pain persists or if it is very intense, it is essential to consult a doctor without delay)
Calcarea carbonica	✿ Eczema of the newborn, itchy scalp and cheeks, accompanied by excessive perspiration
	✿ Spasmophilia (latent tetany)
	✿ Obesity
	✿ Gout in adults

REMEDY NAME	INDICATIONS
Calcarea fluorica	~ Repeated sprains ~ Hypermobility of ligaments ~ Osteoporosis ~ Scoliosis, asymmetry of the spine ~ Varicose veins, weakening of the veins
Calcarea phosphorica	~ Growth problems in children, (emaciation, dental problems, back pain, fatigue) ~ Fracture healing ~ Sensation of chest tightening
Calendula officinalis	*As an ointment or as a milk* ~ Burns ~ Wounds ~ Cuts ~ Inflammation and skin infections
Candida albicans	~ Recurrent fungal infections
Cantharis	~ Cystitis with sensation of burning ~ Large burns with blistering ~ Burning herpes ~ Mouth sores; canker sores

REMEDY NAME	INDICATIONS
Capsicum annuum	◦ Initial stage of otitis with intense burning like that caused by pepper; not better with heat ◦ Pharyngitis ◦ Alcoholism
Carbo vegetabilis	◦ Asthma ◦ Bloating above the navel, aerophagia, gas ◦ Initial stage of whooping cough in children
Caulophyllum	◦ To enable better dilation of the cervix during delivery (in combination or alternating with Actaea racemosa) ◦ Rheumatism of small joints
Causticum	◦ Laryngitis, complete loss of voice ◦ Stress incontinence, when laughing or coughing ◦ Warts under the nails ◦ Paralyzing rheumatism worse with dry weather, immobilizing the person and leaving them in a hunched position

REMEDY NAME	INDICATIONS
Chamomilla	• Painful teething in breastfeeding babies, causing anger, colic, greenish diarrhea, or fever with one cheek hot and red and the other cold and white. The symptoms are better with passive movement (bus, car, train) • Unbearable pain • Hypersensitivity; anger and dissatisfaction
Chelidonium majus	• Digestive problems due to the liver • Hepatitis of the right lobe of the liver • Liver drainage (in combination with Carduus marianus for drainage of left lobe and Taraxacum for drainage of median lobe)
China rubra (Cinchona officinalis)	• Fatigue after fever, hemorrhage, gastroenteritis, or any loss of body fluid (sweat, diarrhea, vomiting, frequent ejaculations) • Intermittent fever • Bloating of the whole abdomen
Cholesterinum	• Corneal arcus (white mark on the iris) • High cholesterol
Cicuta virosa	• Spasms • Epilepsy

REMEDY NAME	INDICATIONS
Cina	• Incontinence, bedwetting (enuresis) • Periodic pain in abdomen and nervousness in children due to the presence of worms • Itching anus and nose, associated with the presence of worms and aggravated at the full moon • Irritability in children
Cinnabaris	• Frontal sinusitis with burning pain • Coryza, rhinitis
Coca	• Altitude sickness: insomnia, headaches, anxiety, respiratory difficulties
Cocculus indicus	• Motion sickness, better with rest and heat • Nausea in pregnancy • Insomnia due to overwork or jet lag • Vertigo better with rest
Coccus cacti	• Whooping cough • Tracheitis

REMEDY NAME	INDICATIONS
Coffea cruda	✎ Difficulty in getting to sleep
	✎ Mental overstimulation with racing thoughts
	✎ Insomnia after good news or on thinking of a happy event (good exam results at school, holidays)
	✎ Hyperthyroidism
Colchicum autumnale	✎ Painful attack of gout
	✎ Rheumatism of the small joints (fingers, toes)
Colibacillinum	✎ Urinary tract infection with *E. coli*
	✎ Depression and tiredness in people who repeatedly suffer from cystitis
Collinsonia canadensis	✎ Painful hemorrhoids in pregnant women
	✎ Constipation with hemorrhoids that bleed easily
Colocynthis	*When the symptoms are aggravated by humiliation*
	✎ Colic (renal, intestinal, hepatic)
	✎ Painful periods, abdominal pain that is better with pressure or by being bent over
	✎ Sciatica

REMEDY NAME	INDICATIONS
Conium maculatum	Vertigo
	Pain and atrophy of the breasts in women who are not sexually active
	Hard, painful cyst in the breast (this symptom absolutely requires medical consultation so as not to risk delaying possible diagnosis of breast cancer)
Corallium rubrum	*When the person has a red face*
	Bouts of coughing spasms even causing vomiting
Croton tiglium	Eczema in the genital area
	Genital herpes
Cuprum metallicum	Cramps from physical activity and in the elderly
	Convulsions
	Spasms
	Tics
	Spasmophilia (latent tetany)
	Hiccups
	Asthma attacks with spasms and difficulty breathing, when the face goes blue

REMEDY NAME	INDICATIONS
Dioscorea villosa	Spasmodic pain as in colitis that is better with extension Sciatica that is better with stretching
Diphterotoxin	Sore throat as in diphtheria, which may be related to antibiotics and Mercurius cyanatus
Drosera	Bouts of nocturnal coughing Asthma attack Whooping cough Bronchitis
Dulcamara	Rhinopharyngitis, the nose is blocked, swollen glands, sore throat, rheumatism, respiratory difficulties—coming on in damp weather, after rain, or near water (the ocean, a lake, a river)
Eupatorium perfoliatum	The flu, accompanied by pain in the eyes that is better when the person is lying down or does not move around
Euphrasia	Conjunctivitis Cold with inflammation of the eyes and nose, with a watery discharge

REMEDY NAME	INDICATIONS
Ferrum phosphoricum	*When the symptoms are accompanied by a fever of 100–102°F, with a pale face* - Tracheitis - Bronchitis - Rhinopharyngitis - Otitis (in combination with Mercurius dulcis)
Fluoricum acidum	- Varicose veins - Varicose ulcers
Folliculinum	*When the symptoms appear before periods and disappear when they start* - Premenstrual syndrome (painful swelling of the breasts, abdominal pain, water retention, headache) - Herpes, cold sores, acne
Formica rufa	- Recurring cystitis with burning and urine that has an unpleasant smell - Excess uric acid
FSH (follicle stimulating hormone)	- Hot flashes during menopause

REMEDY NAME	INDICATIONS
Gelsemium	Fever with headache and prostration, without thirst in spite of fever, better when staying still
	Stage fright
	Anxiety and lapses of memory due to anticipation
Glonoine	Hot flashes
	Palpitations
	Headache with redness of the face and pulsating temples
	Chest pain
	Hypertension
Graphites	Eczema (behind the ears, in the skin folds) with honey-like discharge
	Warts around the nails
	Constipation
	Late periods and hot flashes before menopause
	Prominent scars, as if embossed (keloid)
Hamamelis	To improve venous circulation
	Varicose veins
	Hemorrhoids

REMEDY NAME	INDICATIONS
Hekla lava	Bony excrescences (lumps on a young child's fingers caused by writing with a pen; small round lumps on the hands in elderly people) Osteoarthritis
Helonias	White vaginal discharge Drainage of vaginal mucous membranes when there is a bacterial and/or fungal infection
Hepar sulphur	*In 4 CH potency* Draining pus from an abscess *In 7/9 CH potency* Regulation of pus drainage Dental abscess (take in combination with Pyrogenium) Purulent infection of the ear or sinuses *In 15/30 CH potency* After the drainage of pus
Histaminum	All allergies

REMEDY NAME	INDICATIONS
Hydrastis canadensis	Rhinitis, sinusitis, pharyngitis, bronchitis, laryngitis, with yellow, viscous secretions
	Liver problems with constipation
Hyoscyamus niger	Childhood anxiety when going to bed
	Nocturnal cough coming on when the person goes to bed
	Hallucinations and exhibitionism in the elderly
Hypericum perforatum	Piercing, stabbing pain in an area where nerves terminate (teeth, coccyx, fingers)
	Neuralgia
	Pain after any kind of puncture wound or sting
Hypothalamus	Obsessions
	Feeling of hunger (while on a diet)
Ignatia amara	Spasmophilia (latent tetany)
	Hyperexcitabilty from noise, light, odors
	Extreme emotional reaction causing very changeable symptoms that are better with distraction and worse with boredom (paradoxical problems)

REMEDY NAME	INDICATIONS
Influenzinum	☙ Prevention of the flu ☙ Flu ☙ Tiredness after the flu or after the flu vaccine
Iodum	☙ Dysfunction of the thyroid with emaciation and sensation of heat ☙ Depression due to an emotion ☙ Spasmophilia (latent tetany) ☙ Hyperactivity ☙ Swollen glands
Ipecac	*When the tongue is clean and pink* ☙ Nausea and vomiting, worse after vomiting ☙ Coughing spasm, dry at first and then becoming productive, accompanied by nausea ☙ Asthma attack
Iris versicolor	☙ Burning in the digestive tract from the mouth to the anus ☙ Acid reflux

REMEDY NAME	INDICATIONS
Kalium bichromicum	Rhinitis with thick discharge and crusts Sinusitis with pain in specific places Sore throat Stomach ulcers with burning and pain that does not spread out (remains at specific points)
Kalium bromatum	Agitation in children (behind with schoolwork, night terrors, sleepwalking) with continuous movement of the hands Memory problems due to nervous fatigue Acne
Kalium carbonicum	Flatulence Nocturnal asthma attacks come on between 2 and 4 a.m. Respiratory insufficiency with fatigue, better when the person is sitting down with their elbows on their knees Edema at the inner corner of the eyelids Fatigue Aging

REMEDY NAME	INDICATIONS
Kalium muriaticum	Otitis with fluid
Kalium phosphoricum	Fatigue after mental or sexual activity
	Memory problems
	Impotence
Kalmia latifolia	Violent pain due to sciatica or along the nerves connecting to the spine
	Herpes zoster (shingles)
Kreosotum	Bleeding gums
	Dental cavities
	Foul smelling and burning vaginal discharges
Lac caninum	Premenstrual syndrome (painful swelling of the breasts)
	Migraines, changing from right to left and from left to right

REMEDY NAME	INDICATIONS
Lachesis	✿ Menopause
	✿ Late periods
	✿ Jealousy in people who abuse alcohol
	✿ Tendency to talk incessantly
	✿ Left-sided in all complaints (the patient always has pain on the same side—left-sided migraine, left-sided sore throat, left-sided breast pain, left-sided sciatica—that is worse when wearing anything tight: a belt, a turtleneck, a bra)
	✿ Insomnia with dreams of snakes, death, cemeteries
Lachnanthes tinctoria	✿ Torticollis, stiff neck
	✿ Pain in the cervical spine
Ledum palustre	✿ Insect bite/sting
	✿ Attacks of gout
	✿ Traumatic injury better with ice (black eye)
Lilium tigrinum	✿ Feeling of heaviness in the genital organs
	✿ Cystitis with constant need to urinate
	✿ Hysterical behavior

REMEDY NAME	INDICATIONS
Lung histamine	All allergic reactions, particularly respiratory allergies and asthma
Lycopodium	Digestive problems with gas and vomiting in a person who quickly feels full
	Abdominal distension from the outset of a meal, making it necessary to loosen belt
	Headaches connected with digestive problems
	Urticaria
	Premature aging (white hair, fatigue)
	Impotence
	Right-sided in all conditions (the patient always has a problem on the same side: right-sided migraine, right-sided sore throat, pain in right breast, right-sided sciatica, pain in right testicle)
Magnesia phosphorica	Spasmophilia (latent tetany)
	Cramps
	Painful periods
	Colic and diarrhea better bending over and with pressure

REMEDY NAME	INDICATIONS
Manganum metallicum	- Irritation of the respiratory system - Hoarseness, aphonia - Tremor - Parkinson's
Medorrhinum	- Rheumatism that is better by the ocean - Asthma that is better by the ocean - Repeated genital infections - Erythema of the buttocks, diaper rash in babies - Chronic rhinopharyngitis - Warts - Depression
Melatonin	- Jet lag - Difficulties getting to sleep - Wakefulness at night - Mood problems
Mercurius bi-iodatus	*When the tongue is white* - Left-sided inflammation of tonsils - Left-sided sore throat with whiteness

REMEDY NAME	INDICATIONS
Mercurius corrosivus	Sore throat with crypts in tonsils, white and bleeding, with ulceration
	Cystitis with blood in the urine
Mercurius cyanatus	Sore throat
	Diphtheria, sore throat with a white membrane on the palate, like a veil (combined with allopathic treatment)
Mercurius dulcis	Otitis (in combination with Ferrum phosphoricum)
	Problems with the Eustachian tubes
Mercurius proto-iodatus	Right-sided inflammation of tonsils
	Sore throat
Mercurius solubilis	Rhinopharyngitis white sore throat
	Mouth sores; canker sores
	Profuse salivation
	White tongue with imprint of teeth
	Bad breath
	Loss of memory
	Tremor
	Agitation at night

REMEDY NAME	INDICATIONS
Mezereum	✥ Herpes with honey-like, thick exudate
	✥ Herpes zoster (shingles)
	✥ Itching
Millefolium	✥ Nosebleeds
Morbillinum	✥ After the measles or measles vaccination
	✥ Measles (in combination with Belladonna)
Moschus	✥ Malaise or fainting after an emotion
	✥ Tremor
	✥ Hysteria, nymphomania
	✥ Sexual excitement
Murex	✥ Relaxation of tissues, ptosis
	✥ Sexual excitement
	✥ Slight depression
Muriaticum acidum	✥ Allergy to the sun
	✥ Burns on the skin
	✥ Burning due to acid reflux
	✥ Ulcerated hemorrhoids

REMEDY NAME	INDICATIONS
Myristica	*The "homeopathic lancet"; it facilitates piercing* Abscess, paronychia
Natrum carbonicum	Repeated sprains Intolerance of heat and sunlight, with diarrhea and fatigue Sunstroke
Natrum muriaticum	Emaciation of the upper half of the body after an infectious illness in spite of a good appetite, especially for salty foods Constipation Depression due to disappointed love with withdrawal into oneself Acne, herpes, urticaria, recurring eczema Fissure of the upper lip
Natrum sulphuricum	Chronic colitis with diarrhea Chronic bronchitis aggravated by humidity Following head injury Generalized water retention

REMEDY NAME	INDICATIONS
Nitricum acidum	⚛ Mouth ulcers ⚛ Fissured warts ⚛ Fissure of the corners of the mouth ⚛ Anal fissure
Nux moschata	⚛ Somnolence with tendency toward feeling of malaise and fainting fits
Nux vomica	⚛ Indigestion after excessive eating and drinking (alcohol) ⚛ Somnolence after meals ⚛ Hangover prevention ⚛ Abdominal distension after meals, making it necessary to loosen belt ⚛ Constipation with ineffective straining ⚛ Hemorrhoids ⚛ Hay fever, when the nose runs during the day and is blocked at night ⚛ Insomnia aggravated by worries
Opium	⚛ Constipation ⚛ Absence of pain and desire, insomnia after an emotion ⚛ Somnolence in the daytime followed by energy at night ⚛ Coma

REMEDY NAME	INDICATIONS
Paeonia	Weeping hemorrhoids
	Anal fistula
Paratyphoidinum B	Intransigent diarrhea following food poisoning
	Chronic colitis with diarrhea
Pareira brava	Urinary tract infection
	Kidney drainage (in low dilution)
Pertussinum	Cough resembling whooping cough
	Persistent cough
Petroleum	Eczema and fissures caused by hydrocarbons (gasoline, oil), aggravated by cold
	Motion sickness that is better after eating
	Vomiting
Phenobarbital	Itching, urticaria, pruritus, after eating shellfish
	Drainage after taking barbiturates
Phosphoricum acidum	Depression following worry or distress
	Nervous fatigue
	Loss of memory in elderly people and students
	Growing pains
	Hair falling out

HOMEOPATHY

REMEDY NAME	INDICATIONS
Phosphorus	All bleeding or hemorrhages: nosebleeds, preparation for surgical operations (in combination with China rubra)
	Viral hepatitis with liver failure
	Vertigo in the elderly
	Hoarseness, aphonia (loss of voice), aggravated in the evening
	Pulmonary problems (the prescription and taking of Phosphorus, in this case, are a matter for a homeopath)
Phytolacca	Sore throats with redness (combined with Calendula, perhaps used as a mouthwash)
	Painful breasts before periods
Platina	Spasms
	Constipation while traveling
	Allergy to platinum
	Side effects of certain cancer treatments
	Great sexual excitement in women

REMEDY NAME	INDICATIONS
Plumbum	*When the pain is intensified by movement and better with pressure* ⓒ Constipation with spasms and pain in the abdomen ⓒ High blood pressure ⓒ Rigidity in Parkinson's disease (combined with standard anti-Parkinson's treatment)
Podophyllum peltatum	ⓒ Profuse, liquid, gushing diarrhea ⓒ Bloating
Pollen	ⓒ Respiratory allergies ⓒ Hay fever ⓒ Allergy to pollens
Psorinum	ⓒ Migraines ⓒ Depression ⓒ Itching, skin eruptions, fungal infections (aggravated by heat of the bed and water) ⓒ Parasitic conditions ⓒ Skin looks dirty

REMEDY NAME	INDICATIONS
Pulsatilla	*When the person is chilly but cannot tolerate a room that is too hot and symptoms are better with fresh air* ◦ Colds with non-irritating discharges ◦ Rhinopharyngitis with non-irritating discharges ◦ Red, tearful, non-irritated eyes ◦ Bronchitis ◦ Chilblains ◦ Non-irritating vaginal discharges ◦ Disturbed periods, late or scanty ◦ Venous circulation sluggish, hemorrhoids (better with a slow walk or cycling) ◦ Weeping (better with consolation from someone they are fond of)
Pyrogenium	◦ High fever in an infectious illness

REMEDY NAME	INDICATIONS
Radium bromatum	◌ Rheumatism that is better with continued movement
	◌ Itching
	◌ Scarring
	◌ Following radiation (treatment with X-rays or radiotherapy, repeated radiography)
	◌ For any hair loss
	◌ Asthenia
Ranunculus bulbosus	◌ Intercostal pain
	◌ Intercostal neuralgia (shingles)
Raphanus sativus	◌ Bloating, gas, and constipation after an operation
Rheum	◌ Acidity and burning diarrhea
Rhododendron	◌ Rheumatism and neuralgia worse with stormy weather or hot, damp weather
Rhus toxicodendron	◌ Rheumatism and pain (aggravated by damp cold and better with movement)
	◌ Flu (better with movement and aggravated at night)
	Viral infections
	◌ Herpes zoster (shingles), chicken pox

REMEDY NAME	INDICATIONS
Ricinus communis (castor oil)	✤ Breast engorgement after giving birth ✤ Inflammation of the stomach and intestines ✤ Diarrhea
Robinia	✤ Regurgitations and acidic vomiting
Rumex crispus	✤ Irritation of the throat and respiratory tract on contact with cold air ✤ Bouts of coughing ✤ Itching on undressing
Ruta graveolens	✤ Sprain, dislocation, trauma to ligaments (often combined with Arnica montana) ✤ Ocular fatigue, difficulties of accommodation
Sabadilla	✤ Hay fever with repeated bouts of sneezing, itching of the palate ✤ Asthma caused by allergy to pollens
Sabal serrulata	✤ Urinary problems associated with prostate problems ✤ Pelvic heaviness

REMEDY NAME	INDICATIONS
Sabina	• Profuse periods, painful, with red blood • Genital warts
Sambucus nigra	• Laryngitis in children • Asthma attack with difficulty breathing • Blocked nose • Whooping cough
Sanguinaria canadensis	• Right-sided migraines, and changing from right to left • Hot flashes in menopause
Secale cornutum	• Arthritis and leg cramps • Painful periods at the time of menopause, with black blood and clots • Raynaud's syndrome
Selenium	• Acne • Fatigue and weakness due to overwork • Hair falling out
Senna	• Ketoacidosis in children • Diarrhea

REMEDY NAME	INDICATIONS
Sepia	☙ Hemorrhoids with sluggishness
	☙ Premenstrual syndrome, nausea in pregnancy, hot flashes in the menopause
	☙ Cystitis with *E. coli* (depending on the circumstances, the doctor may or may not combine it with antibiotics)
	☙ Depression with menopause or after giving birth (the subject isolates herself without speaking, does everything from duty not from choice)
	☙ Discolored patches on the face, chloasma in pregnant women
	☙ Eczema
	☙ Nausea on brushing teeth
Serum anticolibacillaire	☙ Cystitis
	☙ Urinary tract infection
Serum Yersin	☙ Prevention of the flu in sensitive, immunosuppressed people
	☙ Treatment of the flu (in combination with Influenzinum and Thymulin)

REMEDY NAME	INDICATIONS
Silicea	Rickets and emaciation in children
	Bone problems: fracture, osteoporosis (in combination with Symphytum, Arnica montana, and Schuessler Tissue Salts)
	Aftereffects of vaccination, especially BCG
	Chilblains, boils, acne, when they are moist
	Chronic discharge
Solidago	Drainage of liver, bladder and kidneys
Spigelia	Left-sided migraine
	Left-sided facial neuralgia
	Palpitations, problems with the heart rate
Spongia tosta	Acute laryngitis in children
	Whooping cough
	Cough resembling whooping cough
Staphylococcinum	Staph infection
	Acne
	Infected eczema, boils

REMEDY NAME	INDICATIONS
Staphysagria	Cystitis caused by sexual contact
	Stye
	Eczema of the scalp and face with itching
	Laceration from a cutting blade (knife, lancet after surgical operations, and the like)
	Mental/emotional problems after suppressed anger or annoyance
Sticta pulmonaria	Dry cough
	Frontal sinusitis
	Colds with blocked nose in spite of sneezing
Stramonium	Delirium due to a very high fever
	Night terrors and angry delusions in children
Streptococcinum	Infection with streptococcus (may be combined with antibiotics, in the case of hemolytic streptococcus)

REMEDY NAME	INDICATIONS
Sulfur	*This remedy should only be prescribed by a homeopath because it may induce the aggravation of certain symptoms.* • Dermatitis aggravated by water and heat (acne, eczema, boils, psoriasis, and the like) • Skin problems alternating with intestinal and digestive problems or with asthma (when there is dermatitis, the digestive problems or asthma are lessened and vice versa) • Stye • Hot flashes in people with congestive issues
Sulfuricum acidum	• Burning sensation in the stomach, with acid reflux • Alcoholism
Sulfur iodatum	• Repeated rhinopharyngitis • Juvenile acne • Flare-ups of arthritis and rheumatism
Symphytum	• Fracture healing • Bone pain

REMEDY NAME	INDICATIONS
Syphilinum	*When the symptoms are aggravated in the mountains* ◦ Bone pain worse at night ◦ Arthritis ◦ Germophobia ◦ General ulceration
Tabacum	◦ Motion sickness that is better with fresh air ◦ Nausea in pregnancy ◦ Cessation of smoking ◦ Cough and nausea with vertigo, aggravated by smoke or cigarettes
Taraxacum	◦ Kidney and liver drainage, especially the median lobe of the liver ◦ Diuretic
Tarentula cubensis	◦ Insect bite/sting ◦ Infections without elimination, with painful extremities, red or coppery to blue
Tarentula hispana	◦ Excitement of unstable children ◦ Hyperactive child who touches everything and cannot manage to concentrate at school
Teucrium marum	◦ Nasal polyps

REMEDY NAME	INDICATIONS
Theridion	Hypersensitivity to noise
Thuja occidentalis	Prostate problems
	Polyps of the bladder
	Warts
	Depression with obsessions
	Vaccination damage
	Cellulite, water retention in lower limbs
Thymulin	Repeated rhinopharyngitis
	Prevention or treatment of the flu (in combination with Influenzinum)
	Infectious mononucleosis
	Lowered immune resistance
Tuberculinum residuum	Arthritis with stiffness
	Dupuytren's syndrome, or retraction of the tendons in the hand (combined with Causticum)
Urtica urens	Urticaria following food poisoning
	Allergies with urticaria
Vaccinotoxinum	Herpes outbreaks
	Herpes zoster (shingles)
	Chicken pox

REMEDY NAME	INDICATIONS
Valeriana	Emotional hypersensitivity
	Severe pain accompanied by spasms
Veratrum album	Very profuse diarrhea
	Diarrhea and vomiting with sweating and loss of consciousness
	Hemorrhages, bleeding
	Drop in blood pressure
Vipera redi	Heavy legs, better when raised and worse when they hang down
	Minor phlebitis
	Varicose veins
Zincum metallicum	Mental fatigue
	Burnout
	Restless legs
	Circulatory problems

Complex remedies

The numerous combinations of homeopathic remedies are called complex remedies. You can, in fact, imagine preparing a complex remedy for each symptom discussed in this guide. I shall only outline a few of them here. Some can be found easily in a pharmacy as prepared and developed by a homeopathic laboratory. It should be understood, however, that it would be best to have a homeopathic practitioner advise you on a personalized complex remedy that fits your needs.

Slimming	*According to your needs, you can choose four or five remedies from this list and have them combined by your pharmacist.*
	Thyroid 4 CH (to stimulate the thyroid)
	Antimonium crudum 5 CH (to diminish hunger in combination with Hypothalamus 9 CH and Hypophysis 9 CH—1 dose of each weekly)
	Anacardium orientale 5 CH (for hunger that makes people aggressive)
	Natrum sulphuricum 9 CH (for water retention)
	Thuja occidentalis 9 CH (for water retention and cellulite)
	Ignatia amara 5 CH (for snacking)

Drainage	*According to your needs, you can choose 4 or 5 remedies from this list and have them combined by your pharmacist.*
(Liver, kidneys, skin)	
	☙ Chelidonium majus 4 DH (right lobe of the liver)
	☙ Carduus marianus 4 DH (left lobe of the liver)
	☙ Taraxacum 4 DH (median lobes of the liver)
	☙ Solidago 4 DH (liver and kidneys)
	☙ Berberis vulgaris 4 CH (kidneys)
	☙ Lappa major 4 DH (skin)
	☙ Viola tricolor 4 DH (skin)
	☙ Cholesterinum 9 CH (cholesterol)
	☙ Uricum acidum 5 CH (uric acid)
Homeopathic diuretic	☙ Apis mellifica 9 CH (localized edema with weak desire to urinate)
	☙ Natrum sulphuricum 5 CH (water retention)
	☙ Thuja occidentalis 5 CH (water retention and cellulite)
	☙ Berberis vulgaris 5 CH (general diuretic)

Vegetable diuretic	Orthosiphon mother tincture (for high blood pressure) Pilosella mother tincture (for weight-loss diets) Lepedeza mother tincture (for excess urine) Erigeron canadensis mother tincture (for excess uric acid) Fucus vesiculosus mother tincture (for weight-loss diets)
Circulation	*You can have a combination prepared from* Hamamelis 5 CH Pulsatilla 5 CH Arnica montana 9 CH Vipera redi 9 CH
Hemorrhoids	*You can have a combination prepared from* Paeonia 5 CH Aesculus hippocastanum 5 CH Calcarea fluorica 5 CH Nitricum acidum 5 CH Aloe 5 CH

Diarrhea	*You can have a combination prepared from*
	🐾 China rubra 5 CH (*Cinchona officinalis*)
	🐾 Arsenicum album 5 CH
	🐾 Natrum sulphuricum 5 CH
	🐾 Veratrum album 5 CH
	🐾 Ipecac 5 CH

Cough	*According to your needs, you can choose four or five remedies from this list and have them combined by your pharmacist.*
	Drosera 5 CH (nocturnal cough, to take for a limited time)
	Bryonia 5 CH (cough ameliorated by rest; great thirst)
	Hyoscyamus niger 5 CH (cough that is triggered by lying down)
	Coccus cacti 5 CH (irritating cough)
	Chamomilla 5 CH (cough without waking)
	Cuprum metallicum 5 CH (coughing spasm that inhibits breathing)
	Spongia tosta 5 CH (hollow cough)
	Ipecac 5 CH (cough causing vomiting)
	Antimonium tartaricum 5 CH (cough with difficulty breathing)
	Lobelia inflata 5 CH (smoker's cough)
	Arsenicum album 5 CH (cough with anxiety, worse between 1 and 3 a.m.)

Smoking	*You can have a combination prepared from*
	Lobelia inflata 5 CH
	Tabacum 5 CH
	Cadmium 5 CH
	Nux vomica 5 CH
The flu	*You can have a combination prepared from*
	Arnica montana 9 CH
	Gelsemium 5 CH
	Aconitum napellus 5 CH
	Belladonna 5 CH
	Eupatorium perfoliatum 5 CH
Sore throat	*You can have a combination prepared from*
	Belladonna 5 CH
	Mercurius solubilis 5 CH
	Phytolacca 5 CH
	Apis mellifica 5 CH
Sleep (problems getting to sleep)	*You can use*
	Coffea 5 CH

INDEX OF SUBJECTS AND SYMPTOMS

Note: Page numbers in **bold** represent principle discussions of symptoms. For specific remedies, see the *Index of Remedies*.

INDEX OF SYMPTOMS AND SUBJECTS

food poisoning and, 203

gastroenteritis and, **171–173**

osteoarthritis and, 84

during pregnancy, 183

teething and, 142, 168

diatheses, 9–12

dilutions and dilution methods, 2, 4, 15–19, 23

diphtheria, 25

dislocation, of joint, **212**

diuretic, complex remedies for, 321, 322

doses, of remedies, 39, 40

double nails, **231**

drainage, complex remedies for, 80, 321

drunkenness, **204– 205**. *See also* alcoholism

dry, chapped lips, **173–174**, **209–210**

dry remedy forms, 35–36

dull, brittle hair, **104**. *See also* hair

ears, ringing in, **92–93**, 217

eating. *See* appetite (excessive); appetite (lack of)

eczema, 61, 103, 132, **147–149**. *See also* dermatosis, of hands and feet; itching

ejaculations, **149–150**, 162, **197–199**

emotionalism. *See* hypersensitivity

emotional/mental symptoms. *See*

also anguish; hypersensitivity about, 38, 44

apathy, **73–77**, 80, 86

with hair loss, 106–107

jealousy, 72, 157, **205–206**

during menopause, 222

overview, 49–50

shock and, **105**, 152

trauma and, 90

weakness due to, 162, 163

enuresis, **156–158**

erectile dysfunction, **197–199**

eructations. *See* flatulence and bloating

erythema, of buttocks, **165–166**

essential oils, 40, 41–42

estrogen hypersensitivity, 194

Europe, 22–23

exaggerated reactions, **193–194**

excitation (hyperactivity), 105, 134, **159–161**, 195

exhibitionism, 161

eyes

allergy symptoms, 61–62, 64

black eye, 89, **230**

blows to, 120

cataracts, **101–102**

conjunctivitis, **114–115**

irritation of, 117, 159

pain, due to physical effort, 124

symptom overview, 45

eyestrain, **164–165**

failure, fear of, 152, 197

fainting, 113, 137

fatigue. *See* weakness (fatigue or burnout)

fear. *See* anguish

fecal incontinence, 111, **199–200**

feet, 126, **132–133**

fever, **167–169**

abscesses and, 52, 54

anxiety and, 71

apathy and, 75

bronchitis and, 94

flu and, 179

gastroenteritis and, 172

with headaches, 214

with pain, 140

sore throat and, 68

from sunstroke, 202

urinary tract infection and, 127

weakness following, 162

fibroma (fibroids), **166–167**

50 millesimal method, 18

fingers, 141, 176, **231**

fissures, **126**, 131, 146, **169–170**, 174, 210

fistula, **169–170**

flatulence and bloating, **56–57**, 113

flu, 124, **178–181**, 325

fluoric constitution, 7

flu vaccinations, 181

food poisoning, 113, 137, 172, **203**

fractures, 83, 145, **170–171**

France, 21–24

fungal infections, 133, **224–225**

gas, **56–57**, 113

gastroenteritis, **171–173**. *See also* diarrhea

INDEX OF REMEDIES

Note: Page numbers in **bold** indicate remedy overview. For symptoms and indications, see the *Index of Subjects and Symptoms.*

INDEX OF REMEDIES